Understanding and Preventing Falls

Stephen Z. Fadem

Understanding and Preventing Falls

A Guide to Reducing Your Risks

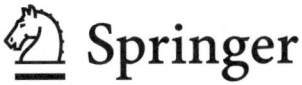
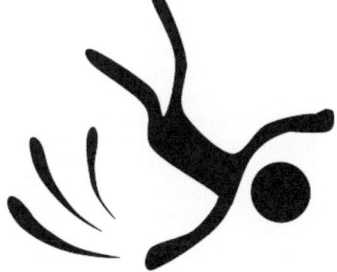

Stephen Z. Fadem
Department of Medicine
Section of Nephrology
Baylor College of Medicine
Houston, TX, USA

ISBN 978-3-031-39154-5   ISBN 978-3-031-39155-2 (eBook)
https://doi.org/10.1007/978-3-031-39155-2

© The Editor(s) (if applicable) and The Author(s), under exclusive license to Springer Nature Switzerland AG 2023

This work is subject to copyright. All rights are solely and exclusively licensed by the Publisher, whether the whole or part of the material is concerned, specifically the rights of translation, reprinting, reuse of illustrations, recitation, broadcasting, reproduction on microfilms or in any other physical way, and transmission or information storage and retrieval, electronic adaptation, computer software, or by similar or dissimilar methodology now known or hereafter developed.

The use of general descriptive names, registered names, trademarks, service marks, etc. in this publication does not imply, even in the absence of a specific statement, that such names are exempt from the relevant protective laws and regulations and therefore free for general use.

The publisher, the authors, and the editors are safe to assume that the advice and information in this book are believed to be true and accurate at the date of publication. Neither the publisher nor the authors or the editors give a warranty, expressed or implied, with respect to the material contained herein or for any errors or omissions that may have been made. The publisher remains neutral with regard to jurisdictional claims in published maps and institutional affiliations.

This Springer imprint is published by the registered company Springer Nature Switzerland AG
The registered company address is: Gewerbestrasse 11, 6330 Cham, Switzerland

Paper in this product is recyclable.

Contents

1	**Introduction**..	1	
	References...	4	
2	**Nonmechanical Falls**...	5	
	2.1 Introduction	5	
	2.2 Nonmechanical Falls: A Deep Dive...............................	6	
	2.2.1 Category 1: Frailty, Cognitive Decline, Neurologic Deficit	6	
	2.2.2 Medications	15	
	2.2.3 Chronic Illnesses and Disorders.....................	20	
	2.2.4 Kidney Disease	21	
	2.2.5 The Kidney and Bones...............................	22	
	2.2.6 Kidney Disease, Weak Bones, and Falls and Fractures	23	
	2.2.7 Congestive Heart Failure	27	
	2.2.8 Atrial Fibrillation.....................................	27	
	2.2.9 Postural Hypotension................................	28	
	2.2.10 Cardiac Biomarkers	28	
	2.3 Conclusion..	34	
	References...	35	
3	**Mechanical Falls**..	41	
	3.1 Introduction	41	
	3.2 What Is Balance?...	41	
	3.2.1 Inner Ear..	42	
	3.2.2 Eyesight	43	
	3.2.3 Proprioception or Sense of Position..................	43	
	3.2.4 Body Sway...	43	
	3.2.5 Being Off-Balance	43	
	3.3 Mechanical (Environmental) Reasons for Falls................	43	
	3.4 Home	44	
	3.4.1 Not Using the Handrails on Stairs	44	

		3.4.2	Slippery Floors and Surfaces	45
		3.4.3	Bathrooms: Mats and Grab Bars	46
		3.4.4	Uneven Surfaces (Jutting Surfaces and Small Steps)	48
		3.4.5	Slips: Wrinkled Rugs	49
		3.4.6	Ladder Accidents	49
		3.4.7	Tripping over Clutter	51
		3.4.8	Not Using the Night-Light	53
		3.4.9	Not Using a Walker, Cane, or Assistive Device	53
		3.4.10	Wheelchair Safety	55
		3.4.11	Standing Too Quickly	55
	3.5	Outdoors		56
		3.5.1	Dangerous Rocks and Edges: No Support	57
		3.5.2	Lack of Guardrail Safety	58
	3.6	Conclusion		58
	References			58
4	**Consequences of Falls**			**61**
	4.1	Introduction		61
	4.2	Types of Falls		62
	4.3	Head Injuries		62
		4.3.1	Concussion	62
		4.3.2	Brain Contusions	63
		4.3.3	Skull Fractures	63
		4.3.4	Hematomas	63
	4.4	Spinal Cord Injuries		65
	4.5	Fractures		65
		4.5.1	Vertebral Fractures	66
		4.5.2	Hip Fractures	67
		4.5.3	Other Fractures	68
	4.6	Conclusion		68
	References			69
5	**Assessing Risk and Preventing Nonmechanical Falls**			**71**
	5.1	Introduction		71
	5.2	Assessment		72
	5.3	Preventing Falls in Category 1: Frailty, Cognitive Decline, and Neurologic Deficit		75
		5.3.1	Frailty	75
		5.3.2	Stroke	76
		5.3.3	Dementia	78
	5.4	Adjusting Medications to Prevent Falls		81
	5.5	Reducing Falls in Chronic Illnesses and Disorders		82
		5.5.1	Age-Related Falls	82
		5.5.2	Comorbidities	82
		5.5.3	Chronic Kidney Disease	83
		5.5.4	Hypertension	84

		5.5.5 Diabetes	84

        5.5.5   Diabetes 84
        5.5.6   Congestive Heart Failure 84
        5.5.7   Postural Hypotension 85
        5.5.8   Sleep Disorders 85
        5.5.9   Arthritis 86
        5.5.10 Vision Disorders 86
        5.5.11 Gait Retraining 87
        5.5.12 Muscle Weakness 87
        5.5.13 Balance 88
        5.5.14 Peripheral neuropathy and Foot Disorders 88
        5.5.15 Bone Loss 89
        5.5.16 Volume-Related Disorders 89
    5.6 Conclusion 90
    References 90

6 Preventing Mechanical Falls 95
    6.1 Introduction 95
    6.2 Home 96
        6.2.1   Handrails 96
        6.2.2   Keeping Surfaces Dry 98
        6.2.3   Using Bath Mats and Grab Bars 99
        6.2.4   Avoiding Uneven Surfaces and Jutting Edges 100
        6.2.5   Keeping Rugs and Carpets Wrinkle Free 102
        6.2.6   Using Ladders Safely 103
        6.2.7   Avoiding Clutter 105
        6.2.8   Night-Lights 106
        6.2.9   Assistive Devices 106
        6.2.10 Wheelchairs 108
        6.2.11 Stand Slowly 108
    6.3 Outdoors 109
        6.3.1   Using Walking Sticks 109
        6.3.2   Footwear 109
        6.3.3   The Hat 110
        6.3.4   Sunscreen 112
        6.3.5   Staying Hydrated 112
        6.3.6   Headlamps 112
        6.3.7   Avoid Danger 113
    6.4 Conclusion 114
    6.5 Outdoors 115
    References 115

7 Exercises to Prevent Falls 117
    7.1 Introduction 117
    7.2 Otago Exercise Program (OEP) 118
    7.3 Fitness and Mobility Exercise (FAME) 122
    7.4 Additional Exercises 125

		7.4.1	Core	126
		7.4.2	Lower Body Strength	127
		7.4.3	Balance	129
		7.4.4	Recovery Step Exercises	130
	7.5	Fitness Snacks		130
	7.6	Soccer and Pickleball		131
	7.7	Using a Trainer		132
	7.8	Conclusion		132
	References			133
8	**Tai-Chi Chuan and Fall Prevention**			**135**
	8.1	Introduction		135
	8.2	Supporting Research		135
		8.2.1	Individual Vs Traditional Tai Chi	135
		8.2.2	Social Isolation	136
		8.2.3	Postural Control	136
	8.3	Background on Tai Chi Chuan		137
	8.4	What Exactly Is Meditation?		137
	8.5	Potential Benefits of Tai Chi		138
	8.6	How to Begin Tai Chi		138
	8.7	Conclusion		139
	References			140
Appendix				**141**
References				**157**
Index				**159**

Chapter 1
Introduction

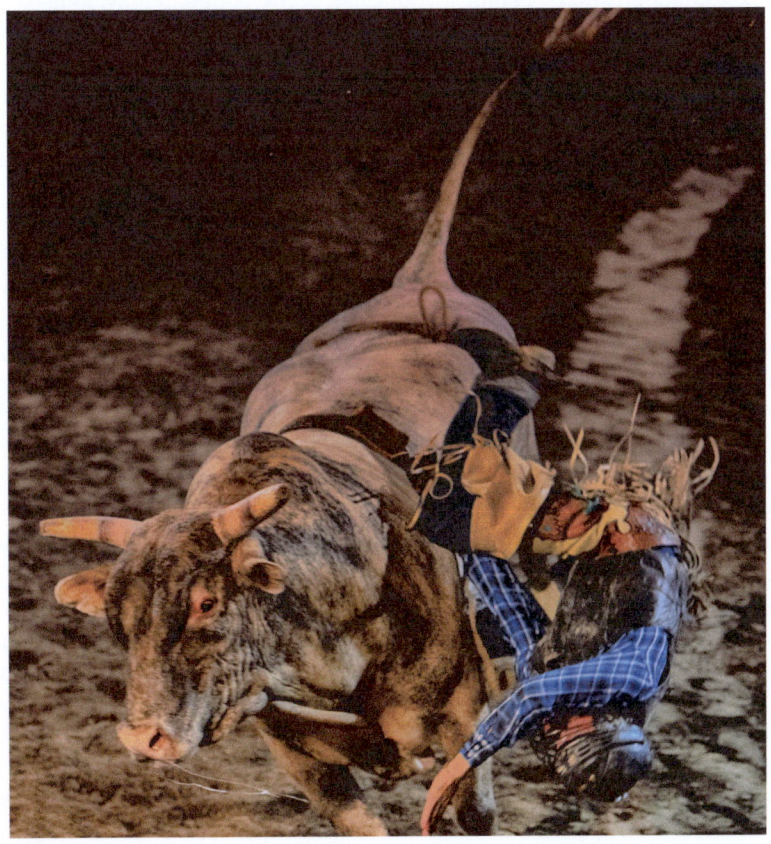

Introduction

© The Author(s), under exclusive license to Springer Nature
Switzerland AG 2023
S. Z. Fadem, *Understanding and Preventing Falls*,
https://doi.org/10.1007/978-3-031-39155-2_1

This book is not just about falls but why they occur, how they can hurt us, and how we can prevent them. Everybody falls. We have all fallen hundreds of times, especially when we were young. As toddlers learn to walk, falls commonly occur but usually are harmless occurrences. Researchers estimate that babies fall an average of 17 times an hour. They are close to the ground, weigh little, move slowly, and don't hit the ground hard. They are padded with 30% body fat and have strong bones. They are already hardwired to know how to break their falls, distributing their impact throughout their bodies, and instinctively know how to grab and bend their knees. Danyang Han and Karen Adolph studied falls in babies, and the most important message from studies of observing babies learning to walk is that they discount the impact of error and focus on improving their basic skills [1]. As we age, we learn the opposite, to consider the impact of error and try to mitigate it. Fear and risks are both reduced by awareness and implementation of precautions. It is just as essential to know how to fall. That is what constitutes the basis of this book.

As the toddler grows to become a youngster, participation in play, gym activities, and school sports also results in falls. Falls are common in gymnastics, basketball, wrestling, and especially American-style football. Impact falls can be harmful, and even lethal, but most athletes do well. The properties that protect the baby—excess body fat, being lightweight and low to the ground—are replaced by muscle memory, developing a sense of balance, strong bones, and well-functioning muscles. Athletes are trained on how to stay fit and how to fall.

As we age, our sense of balance diminishes, muscle loss occurs, and bones become weaker. To prevent falls, we must try to preserve muscle and bone and retain or regain our muscle memory and sense of balance. Luckily, we can learn several useful lessons from sports activities.

One sport, common in rural America, is the rodeo. Thirty billion pounds of beef are consumed each year in the USA, and the skills involved in rounding up cattle and bringing them to market resulted in the development of a popular and competitive sport. The sport has its detractors who have argued that it promotes animal cruelty, but that controversy is not within the focus of our story. In many rural towns, the weekend rodeo is a festive occasion, highlighted by the bull riding competition. Here a young cowboy competes to stay on a 2000-pound twisting and bucking bull for 8 seconds. The bull is exhibiting a primitive survival instinct that is a response to a predator jumping on its back. Bulls are specifically bred for this feature. American bull riding has the highest rate of bodily injury, exceeding amateur boxing and ten times as high as American high school football. Head injuries can occur at up to 15 per 1000 rides, in contrast with professional football, where head injuries occur at the rate of 5.8 per 100,000 players. While an Olympic boxer's delivered punch is 3.4 kiloNewton (kN), a bull's kick is 106.3 kN. The injury rate is around 1.66 per 100 competitive exposures [2]. The bull rider does not know if he will succeed and remain on the bull for 8 seconds, nor does he know his fate with one exception—he knows that he will fall. Falls from an animal account for 48.6% of the injuries that occur [3, 4]. Bull riders of today prepare for a fall by training extensively, wearing protective helmets and vests, gloves, and, of course, cowboy boots. Veterinarians are on-site to ensure that the livestock is handled appropriately for its safety and the rider's protection. Medical personnel are also on-site. Building layers of precaution around the sport decreases the fear and risk of injury.

As we age, our risks of falling during daily activities increase. One out of three persons aged 65 and over and one out of two over age 80 years will have at least one fall per year [5]. If a fall is not addressed, the risk of a second occurrence increases; around 33% of persons who fall will fall again [6]. Like falls in bull riders, falls in the elderly are predictable, and predicting a fall increases the chance of preventing it or reducing its damaging impact.

In contrast to the toddler, falls are consequential at the other end of life. They can lead to injuries ranging from simple sprains or scrapes to fractures and head trauma. Thirty to fifty percent of falls result in minor injuries, but in 20% of persons, the injury is serious and may result in a serious fracture or lethal brain trauma. They are the leading cause of death from head injury in those 65 years and over. A fall may totally change an otherwise healthy and functional person into one who becomes dependent upon others to perform activities of daily living. They may alter mobility and thus impact the quality of life [6].

Falls can be divided into two large groups—nonmechanical and mechanical. The nonmechanical falls can be attributed to an underlying medical condition or the use of medications. Also, as we age or in the process of enduring a chronic medical condition, our ability to preserve muscle tone and balance decreases, impairing our gait and locomotion skills. This too can lead to a nonmechanical fall. The other group is termed mechanical falls. Mechanical falls are related to our interaction with the environment. If we have impaired balance or gait, it makes the likelihood of a mechanical fall more likely. Mechanical falls can happen because the floor is slippery, when we do not use the handrailing on the stairs, or when we trip over clutter we left on the floor. The third chapter of this book discusses mechanical falls and why they occur.

The next chapters are dedicated to discussing the consequences of falls, and ways that we can prevent nonmechanical and mechanical falls as well as their consequences. Special attention is devoted to exercises that can help strengthen muscles and improve balance. Some sports like pickleball have been useful in helping promote fitness and have been adapted by senior communities. Also, we will focus on skills that developed out of contact sports and martial arts such as tai chi. Mastering these skills has been validated as a way to reduce the risk of falls and injuries.

Tai chi is a Chinese exercise that is derived from a martial art. It incorporates many features of both meditation and exercise. Systemic reviews have demonstrated the clinical benefit of tai chi in reducing falls [7].

The book wraps up with an Appendix—and like our own, this is something that we can probably live without. However, in the course of preparing for this book, I have discovered some very interesting scientific relationships that date back in time literally billions of years. Tracing our development on a scientific level will give us better insights into how we acquired the skills we now enjoy and why we often lose them as we age.

Writing this book is the result of a confluence of circumstances—my own aging challenges, a career in nephrology, a specialty that primarily treats elderly patients, and my special interest in bone and muscle disorders and in fitness. Putting in the effort to create a well annotated, readable, and useable book has been a gratifying challenge that I fully enjoyed, and if it can prevent falls, it will have been worthwhile. I would like to acknowledge the support of my family, particularly my wife, Joyce, my best friend and life partner. I would also like to recognize the attentiveness and guidance of the team at Springer Nature for helping move this project from an idea to a clear and comprehensible book. This book is dedicated to all my friends, neighbors, relatives, and patients.

References

1. Han D, Adolph KE. The impact of errors in infant development: falling like a baby. Dev Sci. 2021;24(5):e13069. https://doi.org/10.1111/desc.13069.
2. Sinclair Elder AJ, Nilson CJ, Elder CL. Analysis of 4 years of injury in professional rodeo. Clin J Sport Med. 2020;30(6):591–7. https://doi.org/10.1097/jsm.0000000000000654.
3. Seifert CL, Rogers M, Helmer SD, Ward JG, Haan JM. Rodeo trauma: outcome data from 10 years of injuries. Kans J Med. 2022;15:208–11. https://doi.org/10.17161/kjm.vol15.16389.
4. Butterwick DJ, Meeuwisse WH. Bull riding injuries in professional rodeo: data for prevention and care. Phys Sportsmed. 2003;31(6):37–41. https://doi.org/10.3810/psm.2003.06.407.
5. Ang GC, Low SL, How CH. Approach to falls among the elderly in the community. Singap Med J. 2020;61(3):116–21. https://doi.org/10.11622/smedj.2020029.
6. Wapp C, Mittaz Hager AG, Hilfiker R, Zysset P. History of falls and fear of falling are predictive of future falls: outcome of a fall rate model applied to the Swiss CHEF trial cohort. Front Aging. 2022;3:1056779. https://doi.org/10.3389/fragi.2022.1056779.
7. Geng X, Shi E, Wang S, Song Y. A comparative analysis of the efficacy and safety of paricalcitol versus other vitamin D receptor activators in patients undergoing hemodialysis: a systematic review and meta-analysis of 15 randomized controlled trials. PLoS One. 2020;15(5):e0233705. https://doi.org/10.1371/journal.pone.0233705.

Chapter 2
Nonmechanical Falls

2.1 Introduction

The World Health Organization (SOURCE: **www.who.int**) states that falls are the second leading cause of unintentional traumatic death, causing 684,000 deaths per year. Among those who fall, 37.3 million require medical attention. To understand who is at risk to fall, and why people fall, it is important to distinguish between those falls that are nonmechanical and those that are mechanical.

Nonmechanical falls occur in persons who are vulnerable and have underlying medical conditions that precipitate the fall. Mechanical falls happen when a person who is usually vulnerable, but sometimes perfectly healthy, slips, loses balance, trips, or stumbles. Regardless of the cause, much can be done to both decrease the chance of falling and reduce the risk of significant injury. We are on a continuum of improving and collectively learning from mishaps that precede us. Yet, despite the best efforts of family, healthcare providers, and those who are trying to create a safe environment, falls do occur.

As a nephrologist, a doctor who cares for patients with kidney disease, I have a particular interest in falls because it consistently jeopardizes the well-being of my patients. Many of my patients require a procedure known as dialysis. This is because their kidneys have failed, and the dialysis procedure replaces many of the functions that the kidneys do automatically. A dialysis population is a perfect group in which to study falls, and much of the knowledge we gain from this group of patients translates to the general population, particularly those who are aged. In this index population, age was the primary factor associated with falls, but age alone is not the culprit. In fact, falls are less common in those with preserved cognitive function. Falls are associated with a previous history of falling, frailty, poor nutrition, poor cognitive function, the number and type of medications, several diseases or comorbidities, and decreased walking ability. That is a lot to unpack but it constitutes the main reason that nonmechanical falls occur. We will explain and expand on each of these concepts.

Falls are less common in those with preserved cognitive function, healthy levels of vitamin D, and a normal serum albumin level. The serum albumin is an index of chronic disease. Keep reading for the explanation.

2.2 Nonmechanical Falls: A Deep Dive

For purposes of simplifying and understanding nonmechanical falls, we divide them into three categories. There is overlap; that is, the borders between these three categories are quite fuzzy. The categories are (1) frailty, cognitive decline, and neurological deficit, (2) overmedicated persons, and (3) those with systemic diseases who have trouble with balance, walking, muscle weakness, or eyesight.

2.2.1 Category 1: Frailty, Cognitive Decline, Neurologic Deficit

Frailty

Frailty [1] is the condition of degradation that generally accompanies chronic illness and or aging. It is the result of diminished physiological reserve. Aging and deconditioning vary for many reasons but invariably end in frailty. We intuitively recognize frailty in our friends, loved ones, or patients. It is characterized by poor appetite and weight loss without dieting, fatigue or lack of energy, a loss of strength and muscle weakness, a slowed gait when walking, and decreased physical activity.

Frailty can be rapidly triggered by an acute lung infection, gastrointestinal tract disorder, or worsening kidney function. It also accompanies the end stages of diabetes and heart disease. In hospitalized patients or central venous catheter-dependent dialysis patients who must receive their treatments through a plastic tube, an infected intravenous line can trigger frailty. Frailty can be triggered by an episode of shingles—and we recommend that elderly people, in general, have a shingles vaccine. Influenza and COVID-19 are also malicious culprits that lead to frailty. A fall can trigger frailty, particularly if it results in a fracture or immobilization. Likewise, frailty can result in increased falls. Frailty may follow a cardiac event such as congestive heart failure; a heart attack or myocardial infarction; the sudden onset of a rapid, irregular heartbeat such as atrial fibrillation; or a heart valve disorder. A surgical operation on an elderly person can often diminish body reserves and can also trigger the manifestation of frailty.

In certain diseases, one disorder is complexed with several others. For instance, kidney disease results when the kidneys fail and cannot eliminate body wastes or control blood pressure. The maladaptive responses associated with kidney disease and hypertension damage blood vessels. Diabetes also damages the blood vessels supplying oxygen and nutrients to target tissues and organs. All cells need oxygen and nutrients like amino acids, fats, sugar molecules, cofactors, hormones, and minerals. Over time, when the cells cannot get oxygen or nutrients or cannot pass back the carbon dioxide and wastes that they generate, they simply cannot do their jobs and slow down. Thus, the tissues and organs and the entire body weaken. When blood vessels are damaged by years of a chronic disease like high blood pressure, diabetes, atherosclerosis, or immunological disorders like lupus, they slowly compromise the delivery of oxygen and nutrients to the cell, tissue, and organ failure. This takes its toll. Since this happens over a very long time, training our youngsters to develop good lifestyle habits can preserve blood vessels, leading to healthier and longer lives.

> **The Maladaptive Responses in Kidney Disease and Diabetes**
> Kidney disease occurs in one out of seven people in the USA, and 90% do not even know they have it. 11.3% of the population is diabetic (SOURCE:CDC). The National Institute of Health estimates that one out of three people in the USA are obese. The maladaptive responses of these conditions accelerate aging through various mechanisms, including inflammation. Inflammation is how the body responds to an "attack" and initiates repair. Although its major intent is to protect the body from infection, it is also a response to many other conditions. It can be acute or can be slow and insidious. Its consequences can be widespread, affecting the kidney, liver, pancreas, heart, brain, and muscles. In inflammation, disease states turn on or signal specific hormones known as cytokines. These cytokines recruit inflammatory cells that function like a militia. They are programmed to protect against viruses and bacteria, mainly by oxidation, but when they are too reactive, they also cause collateral damage. An aggressive acute inflammatory response was seen during the COVID-19 pandemic and was responsible for many deaths.
>
> Oxygen is essential for life because it vigorously attracts the atomic particles known as electrons. Electrons are essential for driving the biochemical reactions inside the cells that store energy. This process is done in the energy engines known as mitochondria. When oxygen and electrons do not match up perfectly, then oxygen will try to attract electrons from innocent tissues, damaging them. We speak of oxidative stress as damaging and antioxidants as ways of tying up and calming down the oxidative stress response. Oxidative stress can occur when the necessary process of making energy is impacted or when there is inflammation.
>
> The insidious inflammatory response associated with kidney disease stimulates scar tissue formation or fibrosis. Inflammation damages not only the kidneys but the blood vessels. To understand this better, we must recognize that blood vessels are the networks that allow the movement of oxygen and nutrients from the lungs to the body tissues and carry carbon dioxide back to the lungs. Oxygen and nutrient supply to the energy cells must have to keep functioning.

The kidneys rid the body of excess acid, and with kidney disease, these acids must steal calcium from the bone to act as a buffer. This can lead to excess calcium deposits in the outside rim of the blood vessels, making them hard and stiff. The heart, having to pump against stiff blood vessels, also weakens. Hardened arteries become stiff when calcium is deposited in the outside rim, making the heart work very hard. Eventually, the heart tissues wear out and become replaced by scar tissue. This results in cardiac rhythm disorders and in a decreased pumping ability.

Diabetes happens when either the pancreas does not produce insulin at all (type 1) or produces it too late to do the job of moving sugar into a cell (type 2). The second type is associated with insulin resistance. Patients with type 1 diabetes must have insulin injections, while those with type 2 can control their diabetes with either diet or medications, at least initially. While insulin sensitivity helps the cells to utilize glucose better, resistance does the opposite. The resistance has many causes, one of which occurs in cells when the receptors that carry the insulin signal are blocked. Over time, factors that block either insulin release from pancreatic beta cells or that block its receptor activity result in excess sugar remaining in the bloodstream. The excess sugar directly damages the pancreas, and after a while, type 2 patients require insulin administration for survival. The abundance of sugar excites the cytokines that muster an inflammatory condition. This inflammation also occurs in blood vessels and is known as endothelial dysfunction. Diabetes and kidney disease are linked to hypertension, a condition that raises the pressure inside blood vessels. Hypertension is present in about one of three people on the planet, and this too leads to blood vessel damage. Damaged blood vessels either restrict or block nutrients and oxygen from reaching end organs, eliciting damage. Diabetes and kidney disease ultimately affect virtually every tissue and organ in the body. This damage results in frailty.

Obesity is an energy imbalance that is the result of eating more energy forming calories than the body can use. It is measured by the relation between the weight and the height (kilograms/meter squared or kg/m^2), known as the body mass index or BMI. A BMI of greater than 30 kg/m^2 signifies obesity. Excessive fat intake signals fat cells to reduce a hormone known as adiponectin. Adiponectin is a protein that helps promote insulin sensitivity. Adiponectin also blocks fat cells under the skin from over-absorbing fatty acids, and they instead deposit in the viscera—leading to the "pot" belly. The fat cells not only store fat, but they also play a role in promoting inflammation. Without adiponectin, inflammation worsens.

Sometimes calcium forms plaques or scales inside the blood vessel wall, narrowing the vessels and impeding their flow. They can also form clots and totally block the flow to a vital organ like the heart itself or the brain. They can also block the blood flow to the feet. These are acute and serious problems. Recovery from any such event will likely lead to enough debility to result in frailty.

2.2 Nonmechanical Falls: A Deep Dive

No one lives forever, and we all age. DNA inside the genes of the cells works like a computer code. They code all proteins that form either the structures, enzymes, or the organelles (organs inside the cells) we require for everyday biochemical processes. These strong carbon- and nitrogen-containing substances provide the necessities for cellular housekeeping. DNA codes the enzymes and structures that maintain the mitochondria—little energy engines that drive all the cell's chemical reactions. An intact and functioning cell is necessary for the electrons that create the cellular energy to behave. Errant electrons or dysfunctional oxygen molecules rapidly destroy cells. They work like bleach. They are known as oxidative stress and also shorten telomeres.

Nucleic acids—DNA and RNA—carry the codes that keep us alive. DNA is so essential that if it becomes defective, the body has a way of removing it. Each DNA strand contains long regions of repetitive sequences known as telomeres. These telomeres protect DNA from being destroyed but become shorter as the DNA divides, and as we age, they become so short that the capping proteins that protect the productive portion of the DNA can bind to them. The exposed DNA that is no longer capped triggers the removal of that DNA strand from service; it is destroyed. In aging, the necessary proteins to sustain the cell can no longer be made if too much DNA has been damaged and destroyed.

Telomere shortening is accelerated by the oxidative stress that is associated with errant electrons and dysfunctional oxygen. There is relatively little we can do to definitively stop aging, but we can slow it somewhat. Antioxidants may help protect telomeres [2]. Chronic kidney disease, diabetes, and chronic heart disease all produce inflammation and oxidative stresses that accelerate aging, even if insidiously. Frailty is the response of the body to this aging process and is worsened by chronic diseases, lifestyle indiscretion, and just plain time.

Recognizing Frailty

Frailty may be seen over time in a person because the temples become hollower, the blood pressure may be lower, and the person seems less sharp and aware. It is harder for the frail person to walk, and preferentially, a frail individual may remain in bed. Indifference to life events worsens. When one tries to walk, the muscles may not support them, or they may lose the muscle memory that once controlled the sense of balance. This inability to walk, or even stand, results in falls.

In 2001, Linda Fried and colleagues classified frailty into clinical indicators. She demonstrated the role frailty played as a risk factor for falls. Falls in the frail culminate in a low quality of life and are an intermediate phase between independence and ultimate death. A more recent study established in 2008 classified frailty according to three criteria, a weight loss of over 5% in the past year, the inability to do the sit-to-stand test more than five times, and answering "no" to the question, "Do you feel full of energy?" The sit-to-stand test is demonstrated in this book and involves rising from the sitting to the standing position from a chair without using one's arms.

Fried's classification uses five criteria, grip strength, the speed of walking, the presence of exhaustion, the amount of physical activity, and whether there has been unintentional weight loss. Those exhibiting no criteria are considered robust, while those who exhibit one or two of the five conditions are classified as prefrail. Frailty is defined as having three or more of the five criteria [3].

The Surprise Question

Frailty is associated with a concept known as the surprise question (SQ), where one would not be surprised if an individual dies in the next 6–12 months. The concept has been validated and has resulted in the development of a mathematical equation used today [4, 5]. The SQ is used as a screening tool to determine if a patient is nearing the end of life and will be appropriate for palliative care. In a large-scale study of 21,109 patients with an average age of 62.8 years, 12.4% had a positive response of "no, it would not surprise me if the patient passed away within 12 months." The question was asked by trained nurses. It demonstrated that the accuracy of the SQ in predicting death was 68% [6]. The SQ has been studied in various settings—kidney disease, cancer, inpatient settings, emergency departments, nursing homes, and even pediatrics [7]. Surprisingly, a systemic review showed that the predictive value of a "yes" response is even greater than the "no" response—93% vs. 37%, respectively [8]. The SQ is actually more valuable at predicting if patients will live greater than a year.

Immobility and Frailty

Frailty is the cousin to immobility. This relates to gravity and its impact on vertebrate paleontology. Fish swim in a gravity-free aqueous environment and have small, delicate bones. 365 million years ago, a group of fish opted for land, and at once, these terrestrial tetrapods became subject to gravitation forces on a molecular scale. Among the many adjustments these first tetrapods and all other land species had to make, bone development was one of the most dramatic. The tiny amounts of tension created by mechanical loading led to calcification that followed a lattice-type structure. This structure is mimicked by engineers who design bridges and is a natural response to physical force. Gravity also turned off products that destroyed the muscle so that it could gain strength and support the bones.

The impact of gravity on the bone can be demonstrated in astronauts. During spaceflight, bone resorption increases, and maintaining healthy bones is a challenge space travelers must overcome. Gravity also potentiated the formation of red blood cells. "Space anemia" occurs after just 5.4 days in space [9]. Like healthy astronauts, returning to the bedridden state of immobility leads to losing bone and muscle mass and red blood cell production [10]. While immobility alone does not define the state of frailty, it appears among those with the highest levels of frailty.

Frailty and Falls

Falls are a major health problem worldwide. They are associated with frailty. In a study of 1397 falls, signs of frailty such as reduced handgrip strength and exhaustion both significantly occurred [11]. In China, for instance, they are the leading cause of injury-related death in the elderly and the second leading cause of death in the middle-aged population. To study this, a group of researchers in China used a 40 deficit frailty scoring system to compare the incidence of falls among middle-aged (45–59 years old) or elderly patients who were frail ($\geq$ 60 years old). The study included 13,877 subjects. The fall incidence was 16.6%. Among robust individuals who were not classified as frail, the risk was 13.3% but rose to 21.1% in prefrail patients. In the frail population, the fall rate was 31.8%. The frail patients had a 97% higher risk of falling than those who were robust, and not frail [12].

Stroke

Strokes result from a blood vessel in the brain either becoming blocked (ischemic stroke), cutting off the supply of nutrients and oxygen to this vital organ, or leaking, resulting in hemorrhaging into the brain. An ischemic stroke is twice as common as hemorrhagic stroke, but overall, it is a global problem and the second leading cause of death after ischemic heart disease. Although the mortality rate from stroke has decreased over the past quarter century, the incidence has risen, particularly in those younger than 70 years of age. In 2019, there were 12.2 million incident strokes. Additionally, the incidence of stroke is 3.6 times higher in low-income than in high-income countries.

It is estimated that between 85 and 90% of strokes result from risk factors that are potentially modifiable. The biggest risk factor for stroke is the body mass index—an index of obesity. If this risk factor were minimized, the incidence of stroke would fall 24.3%. Other risk factors are high blood pressure, chronic kidney disease, elevated lipids, uncontrolled diabetes, smoking, lack of physical activity, and an unhealthy diet. An unhealthy diet is considered high in sodium or red meat and low in vegetables, fruits, or whole grains. Alcohol consumption and tobacco use are also modifiable risk factors [13].

Strokes can be either related to emboli, organic plugs that are either calcified plaques, blood clots, or even infectious clumps, that originate in another part of the body and travel to the brain. The emboli block the blood supply to a specific brain area, resulting in ischemia (poor blood supply). This can result in paralysis. A second major cause of stroke is hemorrhage or bleeding into the brain. This can be very destructive and is often lethal. Common reasons for a stroke are atrial fibrillation—caused when the top chambers of the heart (atria) do not pump blood properly into the lower chambers of the heart. There is a stasis or slowing down of blood allowing clot formations to occur. These embolic clots can be pumped through the arteries feeding the brain, causing an ischemic stroke. Calcified plaques that form inside the blood vessels that feed the brain can break off and travel into the brain, locally stopping its blood supply. As with atrial fibrillation, these emboli can likewise cause paralysis. In hypertension, the high-pressure head damages the delicate blood vessels inside the brain, weakening them. They can leak or hemorrhage slowly, leading to insidious damage that may be mistaken for chronic cognitive decline. Alternatively, they can rapidly leak, causing widespread damage to the brain. A subarachnoid hemorrhage can occur when a weak section of the blood vessel wall between the brain surface and its inner cover ruptures. This weakened wall is known as an aneurysm. Trauma can also cause a subarachnoid hemorrhage.

Falls after a stroke are common and have multifactorial explanations. The immobility, paralysis, or weakness caused by the stroke impairs balance and gait. Strokes lead to depression and are also associated with other risk factors like cardiovascular disease, diabetes, hypertension, and genitourinary disorders (including kidneys). The brain is divided into two hemispheres, and they control movement on opposite sides of the body. In other words, a right-handed person with a stroke in the right hemisphere will have left-sided weakness or paralysis. Strokes that occur in the right hemisphere result in twice the incidence of a fall as victims tend to neglect the left, nondominant side [14]. Stroke victims generally fall in the direction of their impairment. This is known as hemineglect.

The percentage of persons who fall following a stroke is variable, ranging between 14 and 65% [15]. It is estimated that 7% of falls occurred within the first week of the stroke [16], 37% within the first 6 months, and 73% have fallen at one year [17].

In a hospital stroke care center in Toronto, the incidence of falls was 24%. Among those who fell, their hospital stay was extended by 11 days. Twenty-three percent of the patients who fell experienced an injury, the majority of which were minor. Thirty-four percent of the falls occurred when transferring; 19% while reaching, bending, or turning; and 9% while walking. The majority occurred either in the patient's room or the bathroom/tub area [18]. Falls generally occur in the midmorning or late afternoon periods and are often the result of losing balance or the inability to sense a cluttered obstacle. This happens because of the gait and balance disorders that accompany strokes.

The risk of a fall after a stroke continues. It is most common in the first 2 months after hospital discharge. But, even a year later, around one-third of patients experience a fall [15].

The most likely candidate for a stroke-related fall is a patient with moderate debility. Those who are too immobile to participate in any activity have a lower opportunity of falling [19]. Caregivers must be trained to handle the immobile patient, however, to avoid mishaps. Falls related to strokes present challenges to caregivers and family members. Opportunities for mitigating the risk of a stroke will be discussed in a later chapter.

2.2 Nonmechanical Falls: A Deep Dive

Dementia

Dementia occurs with functions that are involved with thought starting to decline. These generally involve recognition, memory, thinking, planning, problem-solving, and reasoning. While it can start with forgetfulness and misplacing items, it progresses to the point that the patient can no longer recognize family members, becomes confused in familiar places, becomes socially isolated, and eventually is no longer capable of performing the usual activities of daily living. The World Health Organization estimated that there are 55 million people worldwide who have dementia, 60% of whom live in low-income countries.

The most common and well-known disease associated with dementia is Alzheimer's disease, accounting for 65% of cases. Alzheimer's disease is associated with a type of protein—Tau protein—depositing in the cells that support the nerves of the brain and with aggregates of protein-containing plaques known as amyloid plaques. While this constitutes most cases of dementia, the syndrome can also be associated with the abnormal deposition of proteins inside brain cells, known as Lewy body dementia. This also is associated with a Parkinson's tremor. Frontotemporal dementia is associated with the deterioration of areas of the brain that are associated with behavior control, speaking, and understanding speech. Dementia can also occur as a result of long-standing hypertension, COVID-19, and alcohol. A particular type of dementia—chronic traumatic encephalopathy—is associated with traumatic sports injuries. This list is not all-inclusive, as there are many other diseases and conditions that can result in dementia. At the present time, there is no cure for any of the forms of dementia.

Alzheimer's disease is associated with cognitive decline, and around two-thirds of cases occur in persons who are over 65 years of age. There may be a genetic component to it—it can be inherited. But, its incidence is increasing, suggesting that environmental factors also play a role. It is characterized by plaques composed of a protein known as amyloid that forms plaques. It can also form tangles of proteins known as tau proteins. These help support the brain's housekeeping functions. Risks include the presence of the APOE e4alle on genetic testing, smoking, brain trauma, depression, social isolation, and a family history of dementia. Although there is no treatment, activities that stimulate the brain, a healthy diet, and exercise may reduce the risks [20]. It is more common in women than men, but estrogen therapy has not been helpful in treating it. It is a subject for active research, and many theoretical remedies have been postulated, but the therapy of this disorder still lies in the future.

Lewy body dementia (LBD) is associated with Lewy body deposition and progresses over a 2-year period. It is characterized by the deposition of eponymous Lewy bodies, aggregate fibrils containing the protein alpha-synuclein, in the brain stem, cortex, and basal ganglia. The cortex of the brain is involved with cognitive function. The basal ganglia are involved with coordination and thus are affected in diseases like Parkinson's disease. LBD is characterized by cognitive, functional, and nutritional deterioration and a tremor that is characteristic of Parkinson's disease [21].

Frontotemporal dementia (FTD) is at first characterized by emotional problems and difficulty communicating—including understanding speech and reading, but also speaking. The disease is characterized by deterioration in areas of the brain that control speech and personality. Its course is variable, as are its symptoms. Over time, it is difficult to control movement. In contrast to Alzheimer's disease, 60% of patients are between 45 and 64 years of age. Patients with FTD cannot control their impulsive behavior. Supranuclear palsy (SNP) is a form that is associated with unexplained falls and difficulty with speech, walking, and balance. It is also characterized by body stiffness and abnormal facial expression. It can also be associated with the nerves that affect muscle movement, Lou Gehrig's disease, or amyotrophic lateral sclerosis (ALS), and with Parkinson's disease. The cause of FTD is not known, and there is no treatment [22].

Vascular dementia After Alzheimer's disease, is the most common cause of cognitive decline, accounting for 15–20% of cases. Increased blood pressure is associated with cognitive defects, especially in younger persons. Even whitecoat hypertension and borderline hypertension are associated with cognitive changes [23]. This suggests that we must consider treating elevated blood pressure earlier and more aggressively, as it may be a valid marker for changes in the brain's architecture. There is concern that if the chronically managed blood pressure is too low, it can also affect cognition in the elderly. A large clinical trial sponsored by the NIH enrolled 9361 participants with hypertension. This was the Systolic Blood Pressure Intervention Trial (SPRINT). One of the populations studied was 3250 persons ≥75 years of age. The aim of the 4-year study was to determine if aggressive blood pressure control (< 120 mm Hg) would reduce the incidence of death, heart disease, and stroke. The study was actually stopped early because the results were very good—a 25% reduction in the primary composite outcome of heart disease or stroke and a 27% decrease in death. Although intensively treated patients did have a higher incidence of fainting [24], this large study did not show that cognitive function changed for better or for worse over the 4-year period of intensive control [25].

Vascular dementia can result from various mechanisms. White and gray matter changes occur. Both thickening and fibrotic (scarred) changes occur with long-standing, poorly treated high blood pressure. The high pressures inside blood vessels everywhere in the body trigger mechanisms that cause them to react by forming scar tissues. This decreases brain reserves. Changes in the brains of persons with chronic hypertension can be seen on magnetic resonance imaging (MRI). Since the brain uses a great deal of energy to store and manage the neurological processes that control every aspect of how our body moves, thinks, and breathes, there must be an abundant supply of blood vessels. Some of these vessels are sharply angled to adequately penetrate brain tissues. This angulation makes it difficult for them to handle high pressures. The impact of pressure weakens the walls of individual brain blood vessels by causing microaneurysms or pouching. When these walls rupture, they cause tiny lakes of blood that interrupt some of the brain's circuitry. These are called lacunar infarcts. Over time, this becomes extensive enough to affect cognition [15, 26]. They can result in falls, as has been reported in type 2 diabetics [27].

Chronic traumatic encephalopathy [28] Mike Webster (1952–2002), a member of the Pro Football Hall of Fame, was a center on two National Football League teams—15 seasons with the Pittsburgh Steelers and then with the Kansas City Chiefs. He was nicknamed "Iron Mike," won four Super Bowl rings, and was ranked among the top football players ever by The Sporting News. In his later years, he struggled with mental illness and a personality change, and although he died at age 50 of a heart attack, he was diagnosed to be the first NFL player to have chronic traumatic encephalopathy (CTE) [29]. CTE has since been linked to repeated blunt head trauma and is seen in American football, soccer, boxing, and other contact activities. It develops over an 8 to 10-year period and is initially associated with dizziness, confusion, headaches, and disorientation, progressing to cognitive dysfunction and social instability. It terminates in tremors, speech disorders, and dementia. Patients with CTE can be unsteady when walking and have difficulty with balance. They can easily fall. Webster's autopsy revealed a pathological picture that became typical of CTE, degenerative changes that included diffuse plaques, and nerve fiber tangles, with tau proteins in the thinking half of the brain. PET scans can now identify tau protein deposition and can aid in the diagnosis. There is no cure, and preventive measures are being studied by the various athletic associations.

2.2.2 Medications

As you read this section, please remember that each person is different and that this section is not presented as medical advice. It is for your edification, but the author fully expects you to consult with your doctor or healthcare provider. They know your case far better and can give you the guidance you require and deserve.

Multiple medication use is common. Some are prescribed by a physician, while others are purchased "over the counter" (OTC) or online. The combinations of medications, whether prescribed or otherwise, may appear harmless but, in some situations, can result in the accumulation of toxic breakdown products that can have an injurious effect on the body.

No doubt, the convenience of OTC medications has created value to the public and to many patients. OTC medications are commonly purchased for pain relief (acetaminophen or nonsteroidal anti-inflammatory drugs (NSAIDs)), upper respiratory infection relief (cough or cold remedies), indigestion and reflux (Pepcid, Tagamet), constipation or diarrhea (stool softeners, laxatives, antidiarrheal agents like Imodium or Pepto-Bismol), hay fever or itching (antihistamines), fungal infections (Nizoral), vitamin supplements, and sleep aids (melatonin). "Baby aspirin" has been considered useful in preventing heart attacks and strokes, but it is highly dangerous to use in children. This is ironic since the name "baby aspirin" stems from an era when ASA was commonly used to treat flu and fever symptoms in young people. Acetaminophen is another commonly used pain reliever. Alcohol interferes with its metabolism, creating an intermediate product that can damage the liver. NSAIDs decrease blood flow and reduce the effects of prostaglandins. While prostaglandins are important signals for triggering a febrile response, they also are critical for kidney function and thus NSAIDS may cause kidney damage, sometimes irreversible. In some cases, these medications may be formulated as gummy bears. While these are delicious and chewable, they are drugs and not candy. Even too many gummies can have a cumulative, toxic effect.

The use of OTC medications therefore comes with caution—first, try to be familiar with the label and common side effects, and, secondly, share with your healthcare provider or pharmacist what prescribed and OTC medications you take. They can research any drug interactions that might create a problem.

Multiple medication use is a modifiable risk factor for a fall injury. The use of multiple medications is known as polypharmacy. The use of more than five medications is associated with over twice the chance of having a fall. Some medications are associated with the risk of falling. They even have their own abbreviation—FRIDs— which stands for fall risk-increasing drugs.

For convenience and ease of understanding, we divide FRIDs into three major categories. The first are drugs prescribed for sleep, sedation, or pain relief. These include prescription sleeping pills, sedatives, and narcotic pain relievers. Opioids are included in this category, as are medications used for mental health disorders. Sedation and pain relief may create a state of drowsiness that makes it highly dangerous to ambulate. Not just the hazard of collapsing, but of tripping over stairs or obstacles, or being hit by a car, creates additional dangers. The second group of FRIDs is used to control hypertension or high blood pressure. If the blood pressure is too low, oxygen and glucose cannot supply the brain, causing a loss of consciousness. A sudden loss of consciousness can cause one to uncontrollably fall. The final and third FRID category is the medication used to treat diabetes. This entails bringing the serum glucose levels into a normal range. If the blood sugar falls below a critical point because of therapy, the brain cannot receive enough glucose to power its energy needs. This low blood sugar or hypoglycemia leads to a loss of consciousness and is a fall hazard.

Older people who are on multiple medications have a high risk of falling, particularly when one of the medications used is a FRID. Among 1764 people in the age group of 70–79 who were followed for 5 to 11 years, 36% took six or more prescription medications every day. They had a higher fall rate—nearly one-third fell. When FRIDs were part of their medication regime, the hazard of falling increased 22%. Reviewing medication lists and using fewer FRIDs may help reduce falls. But deprescribing medications may not be enough. Other risks for a fall need to be considered [30–32].

Sedatives and falls A review of articles published in medical journals showed that most people (65–93%) who had a fall-related injury were using sleeping pills or antidepressant drugs. Opioid use varied from 4.4 to 21%. There is 1.6 times a chance of falling in patients taking opioids. In the observational studies, when there was a change in the use of a FRID after a fall, the fall rate decreased. In the elderly, stopping medications associated with falling may not be sufficient to stop falls from occurring and must be combined with other interventions [32]. Although pain itself is a risk factor for falling, pain management with opioids and other sedatives may

2.2 Nonmechanical Falls: A Deep Dive

induce drowsiness. The risk of using opioids is fivefold higher in the elderly and increases further after an injury from a fall. When opioids are used, they should only be used to treat acute pain, and not as the first choice.

Aside from cancer-related pain, arthritis is a common reason for taking prescription medications to control pain. Pain commonly interferes with daily activities but is often not optimally managed. There are many non-pharmacological interventions that can help alleviate arthritis pain. Cognitive behavior therapy (CBT) may be effective. Physical therapy can be a worthwhile adjunct. Optimal management also means managing the medications with the severity of the pain. In many instances, alternative medications should be used for at least 2 weeks before using opioids.

Certain diseases that commonly affect patients can cause nerve pain. When in the lower limbs, this can be particularly disturbing. Peripheral neuropathy is a well-recognized type of nerve pain, and the benefit of opioids for its treatment has been questioned. Drugs such as selective anti-SSRI depressants or gabapentin-like drugs Lyrica (pregabalin) or Neurontin (gabapentin) may be more beneficial and safer. SSRI stands for serotonin-norepinephrine reuptake inhibitors and includes medications like Lexapro (escitalopram), Celexa (citalopram), paroxetine (Paxil), sertraline (Zoloft), and Prozac (fluoxetine). These drugs enhance serotonin, the chemical that carries signals across nerve endings. Low serotonin levels may cause anxiety and depression. They can also worsen neuropathy. The opioid, tramadol, not only helps block the nerve transmission of pain but also helps interferes with medications used to treat depression and generally is not used with these classes of drugs.

When opioids are used in pain management, one must recognize that their metabolism, or breakdown, slows in patients who are elderly. Patients with chronic liver disease such as cirrhosis may also have impaired drug metabolism. Opioids are broken down by liver enzymes known as CYPs (cytochrome P450). In many instances, these breakdown products are then enzymatically changed or conjugated to become water-soluble and excreted by the kidney.

Opioids share breakdown pathways with other prescribed medications, and the use of several drugs that have the same pathways can create the equivalent of a metabolic traffic jam. Some medications block the metabolic pathways of other drugs, creating the equivalent of a road closure. The use of several medications that are metabolized by common pathways can have varied and often deleterious effects depending on the particular drug. Potentially harmful effects can occur with the use of a drug that accumulates when the patient is on many other prescribed medications. Some opioids, like codeine and oxycodone, have active metabolites. Translated, this means that after they have been broken down in the liver and have been conjugated so that they can be excreted by the kidneys, they can still cause sedation and thus falls if kidney function is impaired.

Patients who must take one of the newer antidepressants such as Spravato (esketamine) should be highly cautious of the potential for falls. This nasal spray medication is based on the pain medication and the general anesthetic, ketamine. Its side effects include significant sedation, lethargy, dizziness, and numbness, and it is used for patients with severe depression that has not responded to other therapy.

One of the main reasons why people using opioids fall is that they become drowsy, less alert, and not as attentive to their surroundings. They are more likely to trip over an obstacle left on the floor or to lose their balance on the staircase. Confusion is also likely with the use of opioids. Sedatives like opioids can cause blood pressure to become unstable. Usually, when one stands, the blood pressure self-regulates to prevent dizziness. With several diseases and medications, this regulation does not happen, and the low blood pressure causes a feeling of wooziness or even fainting. This can lead to falls [33].

Diuretics and blood pressure medications Diuretics are also associated with falls. The use of diuretics was associated with nearly a threefold increase in the risk of falls. The reason for this is that diuretics cause the kidneys to eliminate salt and lower blood pressure. The downside of this is that if the blood pressure is too low, fainting may occur. It is imperative to stand or sit slowly and let the body adjust when on blood pressure-lowering medications. As referenced above, the blood pressure self-regulates when one changes positions. Like opioids, diuretics and other blood pressure medications can either reduce the volume necessary to sustain the blood pressure or interfere with the regulatory pathway [34].

Although associated with hypotension and hypokalemia, a comprehensive review of 58 major clinical trials published in medical journals did not show that medications used to control blood pressure increased the chance of falling. The 28,638 participants were followed for 2–4 years. Although there was an increased rate of fainting episodes, treatment with blood pressure medications reduced the rates of death and stroke. The treatment of high blood pressure has more benefits than risks [35]. In this sampling, antihypertensives were not associated with falls in patients (adjusted odds ratio (OR) 0.473 95% CI 0.319–0.700) [34]. In a national cohort study of discharged elderly patients (mean age 77; n = 4056), intensifying blood pressure therapy resulted in an increased risk of readmissions within 30 days, with a hazard ratio (HR) of 1.23 (95% CI, 1.07–1.42). The HR for serious adverse events was 1.41 (95% CI, 1.06–1.88) [36]. The performance and mobility assessment for this population was not decreased. Yet the risk of falling increases when patients have multiple chronic conditions. The risk of falling worsens with excessive antihypertensive therapy because of an exacerbation of adverse events such as postural hypotension, balance and gait impairment, and dizziness. A Medicare claims review of 4,961 patients demonstrated that antihypertensive medications were associated with an 11.6% fall incidence in patients on moderate-intensity antihypertensive therapy and a 10.9% fall incidence on high-intensity therapy. In patients who were not on antihypertensive medications, the fall risk was 9.0%. In a 1-year subgroup analysis of patients who had a previous fall, antihypertensive therapy doubled the risk of another fall compared to patients who were not on antihypertensive therapy [37]. As we will see below, the real reasons why antihypertensive therapy is associated with falls is not due to the medication, but to the population studied. When controlled for frailty, hypertensive treatment is not the culprit for falls. In fact, blood pressure control benefits persons who have a fall risk.

2.2 Nonmechanical Falls: A Deep Dive

Diabetic therapy A systemic review and meta-analysis of falls demonstrated that falls are more common in people with diabetes (risk ratio (RR) 1.64 95% CI 1.27–2.11). The RR of falling was 1.94 (95% CI 1.42–2.63) in those managed with insulin compared to an RR of 1.27 (95% CI 1.06–1.52) in those not treated with insulin [38]. This could be because patients who require insulin are generally sicker and have more of the complications that are associated with advancing diabetes. Hypoglycemia means a low blood sugar. The brain requires a continuous supply of sugar and energy. Without it, the brain shuts down and stops working. When the blood sugar first starts to fall, patients become hungry, start sweating, and feel very poorly. These are warning signs that the brain needs sugar immediately.

In overzealous treatment, there are risks that the blood sugar will fall too low. This can occur when there is a mismatch of insulin and either dietary intake or activity. Continuous glucose monitoring has tremendously aided this dilemma. An opportunity for low blood sugar to occur is the diabetic patient who was scheduled for surgery in the morning and fasted all night. The surgeon had an emergency and bumped the case to the afternoon. Another chance for a serious fall in blood sugar is the patient who is suddenly active. Increased motor activity uses glucose without insulin. Thus, athletes who are not monitoring their insulin and glucose management during strenuous activity can have a drop in blood sugar.

A third cause of hypoglycemia can occur when the patient is treated with antidiabetic therapy without realizing that medications that are broken down by the kidney may accumulate if kidney disease worsens. The kidney plays a role in clearing insulin and increasing sugar's biochemical manufacturing. Coupling this with the altered metabolism of antidiabetic agents or parenteral insulin is a setup for hypoglycemia.

There is controversy over how strictly one should control diabetes in CKD. The HbA1C is a reliable marker for how well diabetes is controlled. Using continuous glucose monitoring, one can estimate the AIC, the estimated AIC (eAIC). This is now termed the glucose management indicator (GMI) based on clinical trials and has a new formula [39].

The KDIGO guidelines that nephrologists rely on recommend measuring the HbA1C as often as four times a year to monitor glycemic control in diabetic patients with CKD. The targets range from <6.5% for patients with mild CKD. This population has very few complications associated with diabetes and is highly functional. Were they to develop unexpected drops in blood sugar, they would have the resources to quickly seek help. Since intensive glucose control is associated with a long life expectancy, it is reasonable that they aim for lower HbA1c or GMI.

In patients with advanced diabetes with many complicating disorders and a shorter life expectancy, there is a greater risk of having low blood sugar with an adverse event than of actually benefitting from intensive diabetes control. Persons in this population may be elderly, live alone, and may not have the ability to seek immediate help if their blood sugar drops. For these reasons, in this group of patients, the HbAIC should be kept at <8.0% in CKD [40].

In patients with advanced CKD, including dialysis, the HbA1C may not be as accurate in estimating diabetic control [41]. Dialysis patients do better with adequate diabetes control (p = 0.024) [42]. However, they have many complications and other diseases that make them fall into a high risk for hypoglycemia. Doctors need to individualize the care in this special population. Continuous glucose monitoring is finding increased favor in the dialysis population [43].

Comment Polypharmacy—using too many medications—may be complicated when patients have mildly decreased cognitive function. Deprescribing initiatives have successfully reduced excessive medication use [44]. Nevertheless, in patients who have many complications, deprescribing alone may not be sufficient to reduce the risk of a fall.

2.2.3 Chronic Illnesses and Disorders

The third category of falls is made of the many underlying diseases and conditions that predispose one to fall. These range from factors that cannot be modified, such as age or a chronic underlying disease. They also include conditions that are treatable. In addition to age, kidney disease, diabetes, chronic disorders that affect the heart and cause lung disease, or cancer, chronic disorders such as arthritis and neuropathy are associated with falls. Living alone, impaired vision, gait and mobility disorders, muscle weakness, and volume-related disorders are also risk factors contributing to a fall.

Age

The older we get, the higher the chance of falling. Approximately one-third of persons aged 65 and older fall at least once a year. Falls account for 70% of accidental deaths in persons 75 years of age and older. They are responsible for an estimated three million emergency room visits and nearly one million hospitalizations annually in the USA. The aging process is universal, natural, and ultimately fatal. Our efforts to slow it are challenging because we are going against the course of nature.

This deserves an explanation because it is a major focus of this book and, no doubt, on all of our minds. Our cells are each controlled by genes. These are made up of strands of DNA, combinations of proteins and sugars that have existed for billions of years and carry the codes to assemble all living organisms. The simplest yeast cells, roundworms, salamanders, and us humans share this basic commonality. This code is intertwined in a long helix. Each of our cells contains around 6 feet of DNA, and given that each of us is a community of ten trillion cells, we contain 60 trillion feet of DNA. This translates to 11.36 billion miles. Think of the DNA like a shoelace with a little plastic cap on the end. These caps, which we refer to as telomeres, can be repaired several times, but after so many years, their numbers wear

2.2 Nonmechanical Falls: A Deep Dive

out, and the DNA frays. The body has a mechanism to remove frayed DNA. Sadly with the loss of each strand of code, we lose some functionality. Eventually, the cells are no longer sustainable, become senile, and die. The greatest enemies we have are inflammation, DNA damage, and cancer.

As our cells die, several events cause us to eventually lose our ability to move and function. Aging can be worsened by inflammation. Also, damaged DNA cells can convert to cancer. Cells and their DNA have the capacity to last far longer than they do in humans. In 1850, the famous scientist, Charles Darwin, visited the Galapagos Islands. What was amazing was that some of the baby tortoises that he encountered were still alive 150 years later. These giant creatures live well—they have little stress because they have no predators, they are vegetarian, they are hardly ever in a hurry, and they take their time breeding. In addition, they have some features that we simply lack. The tortoises that inhabited the Seychelles Islands (Aldabra atoll) were cousins of the Galapagos tortoises that greeted Darwin. A Seychelles Island inhabitant, the famous Aldabra giant tortoise, Lonesome George, died in 2012. In an article published in *Nature Ecology & Evolution*, scientists found that George had genes that handled glucose better. This helped reduce insulin resistance—a cause of type 2 diabetes. He also had duplicate genes that handled cancer suppression and oxidative stress. He also had duplication of the genes that repaired DNA that became damaged by oxidative stress. He also had variant genes that decreased telomere attrition [45].

Since we lack the magic genetic composition that tortoises apparently possess to delay aging, we need to focus on modifiable risk factors to mitigate aging and minimize the chance of a serious fall. Not only are falls a marker of poor health in the elderly, but those whose health is declining fear falling and consequently limit their activities. The body is very efficient and senses whether the muscles are being used or not. Those muscles and bones not in use weaken—that is, their proteins are reabsorbed and recycled. The lack of exercise further increases the chances of a fall. It is no wonder that 90% of hip fractures can be traced to a fall, generally in a person over 70 years old. Many other factors are also modifiable. This means that by understanding an intervention, we can reduce both the dangers and damages associated with falls in the elderly [46–48].

2.2.4 Kidney Disease

The Kidney's Jobs

As we age, our kidney function declines. Most people think of the kidney as an organ that cleans the blood and makes urine. They are correct, but only partly so. The kidney has acquired many responsibilities as it evolved. Freshwater fish always faced the danger of over-dilution and could eliminate large amounts of water. But 96% of fish live in salt water and developed organs to conserve water and eliminate salt. Animals that moved to land developed kidneys that specialized in conserving both salt and water. They needed mechanisms to control their blood pressure. With millions of years of experience, the kidney became a master regulator of blood pressure.

Not just the salinity but acidity in the community of mammalian cells needs to be carefully controlled. The biochemical reactions that govern our tissue's functioning well work only when the acid levels, known as the pH, are set at around 7.4. Too much acid in the body is known as acidosis. Controlling acidosis became the responsibility of the kidney, which eliminated or conserved bicarbonate—an important determinant of acidosis. The kidney also used an ammonia-trapping mechanism to rid the body of acids that were derived from the diet and metabolism. Acidosis is harmful; it turns on mechanisms that break down muscles.

Another job of the kidney is to prevent anemia. As an organ that has a million filtering units and corresponding blood vessels through which large numbers of red blood cells flow, it is no surprise it acquired the responsibility to regulate the synthesis of red blood cells determined by the altitude and the presence of oxygen in the air. Another kidney job is to regulate minerals that help make and rebuild bones. Calcium plays a role in bone formation and in regulating the pH.

2.2.5 The Kidney and Bones

With marine life, tissue support is evenly distributed. But on land, gravity created a challenge—*Elginerpeton* were four-legged amphibian animals that emerged from the sea around 378 million years ago (see Fig. 2.1).

Their ancestors, including us, evolved strong bones for support. Just compare the leftover bones from a recent fish dinner with those of the 11- to 15,000-pound *Tyrannosaurus rex* (see Fig. 2.2)—an animal that terrorized the Earth from 90 to 66 million years ago.

How does the kidney fit in? Since birth, bones must be disassembled and reassembled to grow to adulthood. Gravity creates stresses on bones that enable calcium to deposit with phosphorus into the proteins we know as bone. Areas of the bone with little or no gravitational stress are torn down, so their minerals can be recycled. This requires a complex regulatory mechanism that the bone cell figures out long before amphibians and reptiles roamed the Earth. Bones require several hormones for assistance and control. One is vitamin D [49]—which helps to build bones—and the other, parathyroid hormone, is synthesized by glands in the neck when calcium levels are sensed to be too low. The parathyroid hormone breaks down the bone to liberate calcium.

When kidneys start to fail, they release hormones that eliminate phosphorus. Phosphorus is an important mineral, and despite this effort, it ultimately builds up when kidney function worsens. The failing kidney also cannot activate vitamin D, the helpful hormone that builds the bone and helps the intestines absorb calcium. To liberate calcium, the body maladapts by releasing the parathyroid hormone that breaks apart bone. Since kidney function is poor, excess calcium displaced from the

2.2 Nonmechanical Falls: A Deep Dive

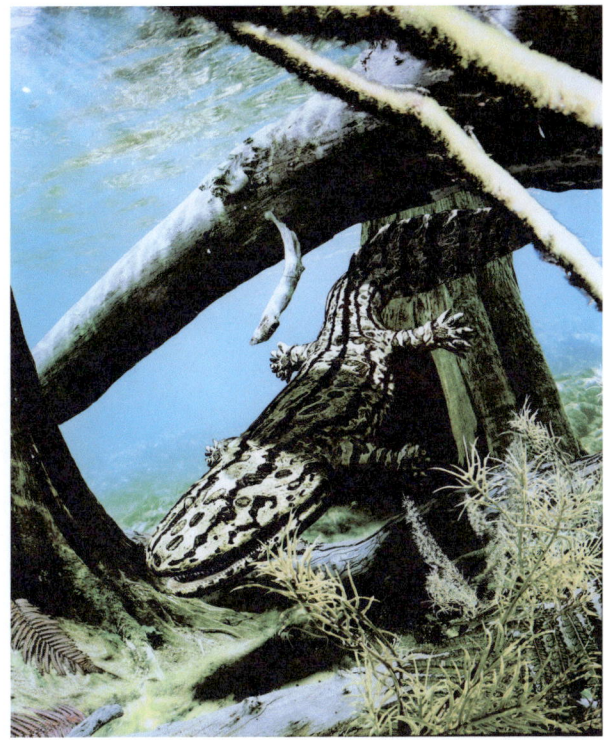

Fig. 2.1 Once the *Elginerpeton* ventured to land, they had to conform to the stresses of gravity. One major change was the emergence of bones that served as major support structures. Photo by Stephen Fadem—from Houston Museum of Natural Science

bone is now free to combine with phosphorus to calcify the blood vessels. The bones become weak as they lose calcium.

2.2.6 Kidney Disease, Weak Bones, and Falls and Fractures

Many patients with chronic kidney disease (CKD) thus have weakened bones and muscles, anemia, calcified blood vessels, and acidosis. Thus, the patient with kidney disease is at high risk for a fall. The incidence of falls in CKD increases by up to 60% with age. Falls lead to a twofold cause of death and hospitalization in kidney patients. The risk of falling is higher when patients have associated diseases like pneumonia, gastrointestinal disease, depression, dementia, or diabetes [50].

Kidney disease often requires a therapy known as dialysis. In an analysis of patients of all ages who fell after dialysis, 28.4% of participants reported a fall, and 71% required hospitalization [51]. One would predict that the combination of a high fall rate and weakened bones would increase the risk of bone fractures in kidney patients. This is exactly what we see. Skeletal fractures are relatively common in kidney patients, around three times as high as in the general population. They are a major challenge [52–54].

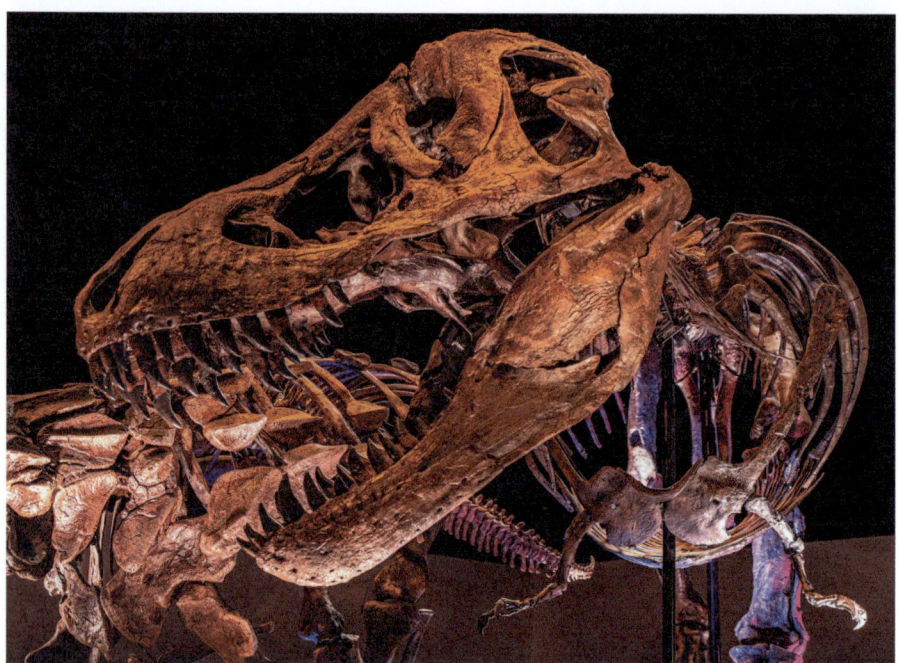

Fig. 2.2 Massive bones support the 11,000- to 15,000-pound *T. rex*. Photo by Stephen Fadem—from Houston Museum of Natural Science

Hypertension

The heart steadily pumps blood through the blood vessel network. This beating action creates pressure. In between the pumping cycles, when the heart is resting and filling with blood, the blood that is in the system still creates pressure against the walls of the blood vessels. If the walls are stiff, the heart has to work harder. Since stiff vessels are also narrowed, they are more resistant to flow, and the resting pressure is also higher. The pumping motion is termed systolic, and the resting motion is diastolic. Blood pressure is measured with a special cuff that is either wrapped around the arm or the wrist. Blood pressure measurements can be obtained at home or in the doctor's clinic. The pressure is read as systolic/diastolic in millimeters of mercury (mm/hg). Normal blood pressure is less than 120/80 mm/hg, and hypertension is defined as a systolic blood pressure of greater than 130/80. These numbers are based on the American College of Cardiology and American Heart Association guidelines. The CDC reports that 116 million adults (nearly half) have hypertension. Many patients are not being treated. Given the risk to patients of heart disease and stroke, this is a major health challenge.

Hypertension is also among the diseases that increase the risk of a fall [55]. This is a modifiable risk factor because hypertension treatment can lower the risk of falls. As clarified above, treating blood pressure with medications is not associated with falling. The medical community agrees that treating blood pressure to recommended guideline levels is beneficial and does not cause fall-related injury.

Sever clinical studies have been performed to look at falls and blood pressure. There are several factors to consider: For patients who are studied in a clinical center, and who must travel, the results will be better than studies where patients are studied at home. This is because the rigor of traveling, parking, and ambulating to a doctor's office self-selects out those who are too frail to leave their homes.

When evaluating the treatment of hypertension in the elderly, it is important not to conflate frailty. As discussed above, frailty is an independent risk factor for falls and fall-related injuries. Yet, a study of 6,595 persons with an average age of 91 revealed a 24.2% history of falls. There was a 20% higher odds of a fall with blood pressures ≥140 mm Hg. When frail persons were compared with those who were robust, the odds of falling were 39% [56]. In another study that looked at 5,236 persons who were ≥ 65 years old, neither systolic or diastolic blood pressure nor the number of blood pressure medications was associated with falls. This was a well-sampled population of patients and looked at Medicare claims. Since the patients did not have to leave their homes for the study, the bias of excluding a sicker and more frail population was eliminated. The study was balanced to assure that racial, educational, and economic disparities were accounted for. The study evaluated frailty, body mass index, history of falls, and quality of life. This confirmed the epic SPRINT (Systolic Blood Pressure Intervention Trial) that demonstrated the value of treating blood pressures to a systolic level of 120 mm Hg [57].

Diabetes

Diabetes mellitus is characterized by an abnormality in sugar metabolism. Its clinical picture has been known for 3,000 years [58]. Invariably, it involves a disorder in the pancreas's ß-cells' ability to either make insulin or to secrete insulin appropriately. It is diagnosed by an elevated fasting blood sugar of 126 mg/dL. A blood sugar between 100 and 126 mg/dL indicates that diabetes is on the border of occurring. Type 1 or juvenile diabetes is characterized by a complete absence of insulin secretion. These patients require supplemental insulin or a pancreas transplant. With insulin pumps and continuous glucose monitoring (CGM), the prognosis has substantially improved. Type 2 is more common and is often referred to as adult-onset diabetes. It is characterized by insulin secretion that is delayed. Since the timing is off, the blood sugars are elevated and potentiate tissue damage. The insulin release may be delayed to the point that it actually causes a low blood sugar level, stimulating the appetite. Type 2 is both potentiated by obesity and leads to obesity. In fact, strict dietary control can reduce the blood sugar and control the disease in many patients. In others, medications can either potentiate the timely release of insulin or block the kidney's reabsorption of glucose. The management of diabetes is a complex subject worthy of an entire discussion that lies beyond the scope of this book. The major message is that diabetes can be controlled, but when it is not, the sugars that linger in the blood and tissues damage blood vessels, nerves, and end organs. Diabetes is associated with vascular disease that blocks the circulation to the legs, kidney failure, diminished eyesight, heart failure, coronary artery disease, disorders of the nervous system that affect blood pressure control, delay emptying of the stomach and bladder, as well as a loss of feeling in the lower extremities, hypertension, strokes, infections, and dementia. Strict diabetes control has been associated with slowing the progression of the disease.

When diabetes is poorly controlled, the risk of falls increases. In studies that evaluated 14,685 people, the number of falls in diabetics was 25% and in nondiabetics was 18.2% [38]. Not just falls but increased numbers of fractures are associated with diabetes. There are several reasons: increased bone fragility, muscle atrophy or weakness, obesity, blood pressure drops when standing, neuropathy, walking problems, poor balance control, and heart disease. The bone turnover is decreased and bone structures are altered. This can be related to the circulation in the bone and the effect sugar plays on allowing collagen to particulate in the bone-forming process. With diabetes, fat cells decrease their production of hormones known as adipokines. These adipokines are important for insulin sensitivity. They also decrease fat entry into peripheral fat cells, and thus, it accumulates in the belly, stimulating inflammation and atherosclerosis [59]. Fracture risk reduction and improved skeletal health in diabetes may be modifiable by dietary control and lifestyle intervention [60].

It follows that patients who are treated with insulin have the highest risk of falling because they have the most serious disease. Hypoglycemia may play a role in falls, and thus the care that people with diabetes receive must be closely tailored to the patient's environment and clinical status—the number of complicated conditions that accompany the diabetes and the ability to respond to a diabetic emergency. Insulin and antidiabetic medications in the oral sulfonylureas class are more likely associated with falls than metformin or some of the newer agents.

The following are newer agents for diabetes control (glucagon-like peptide (GLP-1), sodium-glucose cotransporter-2 (SGLT-2) inhibitors):

GLP-1: These are a class of diabetic agents that also lead to weight loss. The most commonly used are dulaglutide (Trulicity), exenatide (Byetta), semaglutide (Ozempic), and liraglutide (Victoza). These medications are active after a meal, stimulating insulin. They also curb hunger. They have been shown to improve heart and kidney disease. The risk of causing a low blood sugar is small if they are used as single agents [61].

SGLT-2 inhibitors: These drugs block a protein that transports glucose across the kidney tubule, blocking its excretion into the urine. Blockage of this protein helps manage diabetes. It also helps eliminate sodium and can control a feedback mechanism that increases hyperfiltration. Hyperfiltration can damage delicate kidney filters, and hence this class of drugs may also help delay the progression of kidney disease. They also decrease cardiovascular complications. As single agents, they are less likely to cause hypoglycemia. The two well-known SGLT2 inhibitors are empagliflozin (Jardiance) and dapagliflozin (Farxiga) [62].

Chronic Heart Disease

The risk of falls in patients with heart disease is around 60% when analyzing hospitalized patients with heart failure, a myocardial infarction, or atrial fibrillation. The reasons are multifactorial, related to blood pressure drops when standing, abnormal heart conduction, and structural heart disease being most likely to cause falls.

2.2.7 Congestive Heart Failure

Structural heart disease may include a weak cardiac muscle, known as a cardiomyopathy, or an abnormally functioning heart valve. Since the heart must constantly move blood between chambers to ensure it is well oxygenated in the lungs and delivered to all tissues, valves are necessary to ensure that blood is not pumped back into either the upper chambers when the ventricle contracts or the ventricle itself, when it relaxes and fills. The valves ensure that blood will always move forward but may leak. Heart failure increases the odds of falling by 14% in the elderly, and those with a heart failure diagnosis have a fourfold increased risk of fracturing a hip or limb compared with those of other heart disease. The American Heart Association (AHA) has developed a consensus statement that encompasses falls. They suggest that an interdisciplinary approach is needed to decrease these risks.

2.2.8 Atrial Fibrillation

Atrial fibrillation is a condition where the upper chambers of the heart pump erratically and do not send regular signals to the lower chambers of the heart. Therefore, the pumping action of the heart is sporadic and irregular. Not only does this lead to a decreased cardiac output of blood containing essential nutrients and oxygen, but the slowed blood flow in the upper chambers leads to blood clots that can pass through the heart and into the brain, causing a stroke [63].

Atrial fibrillation doubles the risk of falling. It is common in the elderly but also occurs in younger people who have intrinsic conduction disorders. The heart systematically sends signals from the sinus node to the atrioventricular (AV) node and then distributes them through the His-Purkinje system throughout the heart. A block in the AV node is associated with an increased risk of atrial fibrillation and ventricular arrhythmia. This is actually a misnomer. There is not a true block in the AV node but a delay. This delay may be related to fibrosis, medications, or reversible disorders such as thyroid disease. A first-degree AV block is considered benign, but is a predictor of severe arrhythmias, and associated with a higher placement of pacemakers and implantable defibrillators. It is associated with a higher mortality rate [64, 65].

Atrial fibrillation can also be associated with acute disorders like COVID-19 [66]. It has multiple etiologies and thus is linked to illnesses like chronic kidney disease. The accumulation of uremic toxins can cause oxidative injury and damage the structure of the AV node. Anemia increases the workload of the heart. Inflammation can lead to damage to the AV node's structure and can cause fibrosis. Kidney disease is associated with derangements of minerals that the kidney is responsible for eliminating, particularly those involved with electrical conduction such as potassium and calcium and with magnesium which is essential for energy since it is bound to ATP. Since the conduction system relies on the conversion of chemicals to electricity, it is very sensitive to changes to all of these minerals.

The initial blood thinning agent used to prevent atrial clot formation and strokes was difficult to control and has been replaced by newer agents that target different clotting factors and are safer to use. Medications can be used to control the heart rate, but the best therapies are either an ablation of some of the excitatory areas that are causing the irregular heartbeat or the Watchman implant. The ablation therapy, while successful, still requires that the majority of patients continue taking a blood thinner.

2.2.9 Postural Hypotension

When changing from a lying to a sitting or sitting to standing position, one may become dizzy. This may be related to a decrease in blood pressure. Orthostatic and postural hypotension are terms used to describe this condition. It is characterized by a 20 mm Hg or more drop in blood pressure with position changes. It may be related to the nerve damage that is associated with diabetes or could be secondary to diuretics used to treat congestive heart failure or hypertension. Patients who are unable to safely stand are at a high risk for a fall. Managing the underlying causes starts with adjusting medications, wearing compression garments, and avoiding environments that can potentiate the problem. Occasionally, medications are used to control postural hypotension.

2.2.10 Cardiac Biomarkers

Biomarkers are molecules that can be detected after some biological event. They are leftover reminders that something happened. As science advances, we discover more and more biomarkers that help us with early and accurate disease detection. One such biomarker is troponin. Troponin is part of the heart muscle contraction system and helps to tie the two muscle filaments, actin and myosin, together when the heart is stimulated to contract. Troponin levels can be elevated for various reasons, including endurance exercise and chronic kidney disease. They are frequently associated with acute myocardial infarction. In a population of patients with an average age of 75 who fell, 22.5% of men had an elevated troponin level, suggesting that it might have value in predicting the potential for a fall in older men [67].

Chronic Lung Diseases

Chronic obstructive pulmonary disease (COPD) is most commonly called emphysema. It is most common in persons who have smoked cigarettes. A review of what is known in the medical literature demonstrated that the fall rate in COPD was 30%. Twenty-four percent fell frequently. Age, smoking, a previous history of falls, coronary artery disease, using supplemental oxygen, impaired balance, and the number of medications and coexisting medical problems all contributed to the risks of falls. Females with lung disease fell more frequently than men [68].

In addition to intrinsic lung deterioration, patients with lung disease have chronic inflammation, muscle weakness, and alterations in how their nerves interact with muscles. Using biomechanics, scientists have studied the posture of patients with COPD. Although swaying is normal when standing, COPD patients have greater amounts of sway. This is more intense when patients close their eyes or stand on an unstable surface like foam. This may respond to therapy. The speed of one's gait is a predictor of falling. COPD patients have a slower gait as their disease progresses. These changes are supplemental to gait disturbances and poor utilization of oxygen [69].

Sleep Disorders and Falls

It is common for older people to have trouble both falling asleep and sleeping throughout the night. This may be related to other medical problems like heart disease, medications, and lifestyle changes such as a lack of exercise. Also, our body has a 24-hour cycle biological clock that is controlled by the brain and synchronized to the hour of the day and levels of an internal sleep hormone known as melatonin. Our melatonin levels decrease as we age. In some people, the circadian rhythm may be altered to the extent that people are sleepless at night and sleep excessively during the day. Older women are more likely to experience sleep disorders. Sleep disorders can cause a risk of falling [70]. Excessive daytime sleeping is independently associated with falls in women, and these falls are more likely to occur outside [71].

Cognitive behavioral therapy may help persons with sleep disorders, but spending excessive time in bed and not having a regular sleep schedule can aggravate a sleep disorder. Persons are advised to get out of bed when unable to fall asleep. Napping and lack of exercise, spending less time outdoors, avoiding sunshine, and drinking caffeine or alcohol in the evening are well known to affect sleep [72].

Cancer and Chronic Conditions

Many patients have trouble with walking, balance, muscle strength, or eyesight due to the complications of a chronic disease that they endure. It is well established that they are at risk for a fall. Add aging and disability to chronic disease, and the risk of a fall worsens. A study of 79 consecutive admissions to intermediate care facilities was performed in 1986. It showed that 25 patients fell recurrently. Fall risks were characterized by the ability to walk, bear weight, hear, and see adequately. One's morale and mental status contribute to the risk. Back disorders, drops in blood pressure when standing, and the number of medications one was taking also played a role. Falls were also related to the ability to perform daily, routine activities. The risks added up. In those patients who had seven or more factors, the chance of falling was 100%. Around a third of the patients who had four to six risk factors fall. The fall risk was not identified in persons with less than three risk factors. Tests that demonstrated walking ability were the best predictor of recurrent falling [73].

Surviving a serious illness such as cancer is a major challenge. It is emotionally wrenching—a roller coaster of emotional highs and lows. It often entails surgical procedures, chemotherapy, radiation therapy, pain management, and rehabilitation or reconstruction. Many cancer survivors have physical limitations resulting from removing vital tissue or therapy to a diseased organ or limb. Persons adapt to having experienced an illness like cancer based on individual traits and features, but nearly all persons who sustain a serious malignancy are left with emotional remembrances that affect their lives. If we are fortunate, we can gain from the painful experiences of being ill and develop a stronger sense of compassion for fellow human beings [74].

The site of a tumor and how advanced it became when arrested determines the residual defects, if any. Many very serious cancers are successfully treated and do not physically impair the patient. Others who are less fortunate are left with impairments that can result in a fall. In fact, many cancer survivors have a high risk of a fall. The risk of falling is related to the ability to perform daily activities. Persons who fall once are likely to fall a second time. This fall risk is not necessarily related to age and can occur in any age group. Evidence to support the risks of a fall trended recurrently through several quality medical journal articles. These included medication type, the ability to walk or balance, and cognitive and physical ability [75].

Arthritis and Peripheral Neuropathy

The odds of falling increase with osteoarthritis, depending on the number of joints involved. A longitudinal study of men and women over 45 years old in rural North Carolina determined that the odds of falling when one joint is involved are 53%, 74 with two joints, and 85% with three to four joints. Arthritis involving the knee or hip is associated with increased odds of falling [76].

Living Alone

The English Longitudinal Study of Aging is a national study of people over the age of 50 living in private households in England. A review of fall incidences from self-reports and hospitalizations revealed that 52% of people self-reported having fallen. Fewer than 10% had a fall-related hospitalization. There was a 17% risk of falls among individuals who lived alone. In the hospital group, the risk of falling was 29% [77]. This study did not distinguish which patients had CKD.

Vision Disorders

The risk of falling in 251 persons with a visual impairment aged 65–92 years was examined. There were nearly 600 falls during a year period. Smoking, awakening at night, and having glaucoma or retinal degeneration increased the risk of falls [78]. In addition to visual acuity, the inability to accurately judge depth perception, or having an impairment, also increased the fall risk [79].

Gait, Balance, and Mobility Disorders

Balance is controlled by vision, sensations from the inner part of the ear, and how we perceive our position using our joints and muscles. Falls result from underlying diseases and conditions affecting balance, gait, and mobility. Kidney disease is an example a fall risk that may affect balance, gait, and mobility. Advancing age and living alone without social support increase the risk of falling and subsequently injuring oneself. Impaired vision may increase the susceptibility to falling. An acute inner ear disorder can also affect balance and lead to falls. Clinical fall conditions include hypertension, diabetes, cardiovascular disease, and arthritis. Primary or secondary disorders affecting the nerves can be related to diabetes, medications, or a disorder known as amyloidosis. These can cause falls. Acute conditions that relate to volume depletion, such as dehydration secondary to poor fluid intake, over-diuresis, vomiting, or diarrhea, may result in postural hypotension. This list of disease states highlights conditions that can precede a fall but are not inclusive.

Normally we sway slightly when standing. However, in those who are elderly or at risk of falling, this sway is exaggerated [80].

Gait disorders stem from various clinical disorders and, in the aging population, are associated with higher fall risks. The assessment of gait is part of the standard neurological evaluation. Inspection of walking patterns may reveal a neurological disorder (stroke, Parkinson's disease, ataxia, spasticity, and frontal gait) or a non-neurological disturbance related to arthritis or peripheral vascular disease. Ataxic gaits are generally wide-based and unsteady. They are associated with poor balance. Gait disorders may be associated with neuropathy and loss of sensation, foot drop, and decreased reflexes. Patients with a frontal gait have a wide base, take short strips, and have difficulty lifting their feet. The patient with a Parkinsonian gait may take small, shuffling, jerky steps and festinate with a quick, short stride. They may not swing their arms when walking. Spasticity may be associated with scissoring, crossing one leg in front of another when walking. A proximal myopathy may be associated with a waddling gait [81]. In a study of 632 elderly patients with gait disorders, the fall rate was 39% (244 subjects). The average age of participants was 80.6 years of age. Neurologic gait disorders were more frequently associated with a slower gait velocity. Falls were associated with moderately severe neurological gaits [82].

Studies of the gait of older adults who fall reveal that they have a more constrained, less adaptable trunk movement compared to younger people and that the walking pattern is different from those who do not fall [83]. Other studies have demonstrated that while a decreased walking speed was not associated with falls, a decreased stride length was associated with falls in men over 74 years of age [84].

Muscle Weakness

Muscle breakdown and production should always be in balance. When breakdown exceeds production, the muscles weaken. This is known as sarcopenia. CKD is among the disorders that potentiate the breakdown of muscle. Other disorders include a lack of activity, space travel, inflammatory diseases such as cancer or HIV, severe infections, starvation, and metabolic acidosis. Sarcopenia is also associated with advancing age and diabetes [85, 86]. Vitamin D deficiency and the inability to properly utilize insulin also accelerate muscle loss. Sarcopenia is a major risk for falls. A review of clinical studies in medical journals included 52,838 persons who were either 65 years of age or older. Almost half of the studies reported a significantly higher risk of falls and fractures in persons with sarcopenia [87]. Sarcopenia also appears to play a role in frailty [88].

Bone Loss

As mentioned above, our bones are the response to living in a gravity-driven environment. Bone develops when calcium deposits in connective tissue. The bones support the body and are essential for locomotion. Therefore, they must have the ability to adapt their structure to environmental stresses. This adaptation is known as bone remodeling. The bone that is not used for support is resorbed by a group of cells known as osteoclasts. Osteoclasts also play a role in disease states like osteoporosis and cancer.

A bone cell that makes bone is called an osteoblast. The osteoblast begins its life as a stem cell. Bone-making proteins are better known as bone morphogenic proteins (BMPs). They induce the stem cells to become osteoblasts. BMPs are turned on by gravity through compression. This action turns on a master gene to make a protein with a very catchy name—Runx2. Runx2 sends signals that tell DNA to turn on a specific patch of RNA to make the matrix that will become bone. Runx2 is a transcription factor [89]. Genes work when their DNA is signaled by transcription factors like Runx2 to incorporate RNA to send code to the areas of the cells that produce proteins [90]. The

2.2 Nonmechanical Falls: A Deep Dive

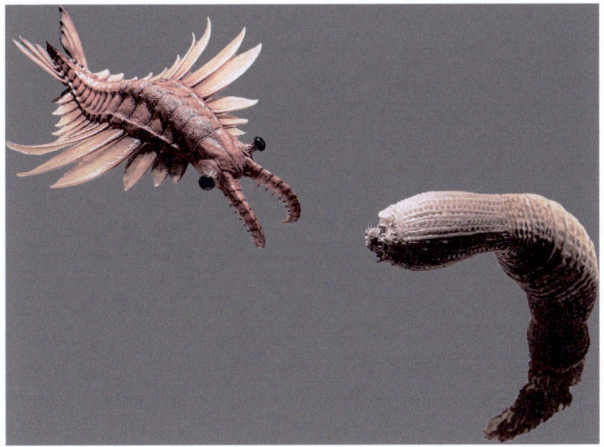

Fig. 2.3 Calcified organisms from millions of years ago taught us the basics of depositing calcium into collagen to create shells and then teeth and bones. Photography by Stephen Fadem. From the Houston Museum of Natural Science

proteins produced are all essential for capturing calcium, work in complex unison, and developed this mechanism 541 million years ago (see Fig. 2.3). The major protein is collagen, and along with neighboring proteins, it creates the collagen-containing matrix within which calcium resides. Among the hormones that control bone formation, parathyroid hormone is chiefly responsible for bone breakdown or resorption. Bone formation and mineralization are complex, and a reflection on health and well-being.

Osteoporosis is the imbalance between bone formation and breakdown. The breakdown of bone is associated with an inflammatory molecule nuclear factor-κß (NF-κß). Osteoporosis is measured by the bone mineral density (BMD) test which indexes the amount of dense mineral in the bone. It is a global health issue. The lifetime probability of sustaining a fracture related to osteoporosis in postmenopausal European woman has been estimated at 40% [91]. It is worsened by the use of corticosteroids and improved with the use of estrogens. Smoking and alcohol consumption, a family history, advancing age especially being postmenopause for women, a lack of exercise, and poor nutrition are closely associated with decreased mineralization of the bone. It is seen in several chronic disorders, including kidney and liver disease, inflammatory bowel disease, celiac disease, anorexia nervosa, rheumatoid arthritis, and type 1 diabetes [92]. Vitamin D is integral to bone development and growth, even as we age. Estrogens are also critical for bone maintenance. As women age past menopause, lower estrogen levels are a major reason for osteoporosis [93, 94].

A side effect of falls associated with osteoporosis is a fractured hip. Hip fractures have a high mortality rate. In a Norwegian study of 146,132 people, 24.3% died within the first year. But, within the first 30 days, the fall causing the fracture was the underlying cause in over half the cases [95].

It is a well-known fact that space travel causes bone loss and that gravity is essential for bone formation. Muscles are also essential. As babies learn to crawl, their core muscles are not strong enough for them to walk upright. After a few months, they are able to do so. As they continue to walk, the bones that bear the pressure of walking grow along stress lines. As we age we lose muscles, and the core muscles that support our upright posture become weak. The lack of mobility also contributes to weakened bones. Osteosarcopenia is the combined syndrome of decreased muscle protein synthesis and of new bone formation. It is characteristic of aging, making persons prone to falls. In addition, falls in patients with osteosarcopenia are more likely to result in a fracture.

Volume-Related Disorders

When one does not consume enough fluid, the blood pressure can fall, the skin becomes dry, and one becomes thirsty. Dehydration can result from inadequate water intake, lack of access to water, vomiting, or diarrhea. Exercising, running, or hiking without replenishing the water losses associated with exercise and the hot sun can lead to severe dehydration and even heat exhaustion. The kidney tries to retain water and salt—and this is reflected in the blood tests—the blood urea nitrogen (BUN), a kidney test, rises as does the serum sodium level. A study of health records from the University of Wisconsin identified 11,622 dehydrated patients. Among these, the odds ratio of a fall statistically rose with dehydration. Dehydration was also associated with antipsychotic medications and loop diuretics [96].

The dialysis procedure that is used to clean the blood of patients with advanced kidney disease may cause a drop in the blood pressure and stress on the heart. This stress can be related to a sudden lowering in body fluids, low oxygen levels, an irregular heartbeat, and electrolyte abnormalities [97]. In addition to the adverse consequences of stress related to dialysis treatments, some dialysis patients may have sudden drops in blood pressure when standing. This is called orthostatic hypotension and is particularly true in diabetes because the autonomic or involuntary nervous system cannot regulate blood pressure when one stands. Standing and then walking unassisted when orthostatic hypotension is present may result in a post-dialysis fall. It was reported that while 34.8% of patients may have orthostatic hypotension predialysis, 69.6% have orthostatic hypotension after treatment. The underlying cardiac stress of dialysis, the use of blood pressure-lowering medications, autonomic insufficiency, and excessive amounts of fluid gained between dialysis treatments predispose patients to postural hypotension and the risk of falling [98].

2.3 Conclusion

Nonmechanical falls are associated with medical illnesses. They can be categorized into falls related to cognitive disorders or strokes, falls secondary to medication, and falls that are associated with other clinical conditions like diabetes, heart and kidney disease, or disorders of gait or balance. Patients should discuss the risk of falling with their doctors and take the necessary measures to decrease the chances of a fall or injury. In the next chapter, we will discuss the different types of mechanical falls.

References

1. Cheng MH, Chang SF. Frailty as a risk factor for falls among community dwelling people: evidence from a meta-analysis. J Nurs Scholarsh. 2017;49(5):529–36. https://doi.org/10.1111/jnu.12322.
2. Xu Q, Parks CG, DeRoo LA, Cawthon RM, Sandler DP, Chen H. Multivitamin use and telomere length in women. Am J Clin Nutr. 2009;89(6):1857–63. https://doi.org/10.3945/ajcn.2008.26986.
3. Fried LP, Tangen CM, Walston J, Newman AB, Hirsch C, Gottdiener J, et al. Frailty in older adults: evidence for a phenotype. J Gerontol A Biol Sci Med Sci. 2001;56(3):M146–56. https://doi.org/10.1093/gerona/56.3.m146.
4. Downar J, Goldman R, Pinto R, Englesakis M, Adhikari NK. The "surprise question" for predicting death in seriously ill patients: a systematic review and meta-analysis. CMAJ. 2017;189(13):E484–e93. https://doi.org/10.1503/cmaj.160775.
5. Gaffney L, Jonsson A, Judge C, Costello M, O'Donnell J, O'Caoimh R. Using the "surprise question" to predict frailty and healthcare outcomes among older adults attending the emergency department. Int J Environ Res Public Health. 2022;19(3) https://doi.org/10.3390/ijerph19031709.
6. Yen Y-F, Lee Y-L, Hu H-Y, Sun W-J, Ko M-C, Chen C-C, et al. Early palliative care: the surprise question and the palliative care screening tool—better together. BMJ Support Palliat Care. 2022;12(2):211–7. https://doi.org/10.1136/bmjspcare-2019-002116.
7. Jennings KS, Marks S, Lum HD. The surprise question as a prognostic tool #360. J Palliat Med. 2018;21(10):1529–30. https://doi.org/10.1089/jpm.2018.0348.
8. White N, Kupeli N, Vickerstaff V, Stone P. How accurate is the 'Surprise Question' at identifying patients at the end of life? A systematic review and meta-analysis. BMC Med. 2017;15(1):139. https://doi.org/10.1186/s12916-017-0907-4.
9. Trudel G, Shafer J, Laneuville O, Ramsay T. Characterizing the effect of exposure to microgravity on anemia: more space is worse. Am J Hematol. 2020;95(3):267–73. https://doi.org/10.1002/ajh.25699.
10. Minaire P. Immobilization osteoporosis: a review. Clin Rheumatol. 1989;8(Suppl 2):95–103. https://doi.org/10.1007/bf02207242.
11. Duarte GP, Santos JLF, Lebrão ML, Duarte YAO. Relationship of falls among the elderly and frailty components. Rev Bras Epidemiol. 2019;21(Suppl 02):e180017. https://doi.org/10.1590/1980-549720180017.supl.2.
12. Lu Z, Er Y, Zhan Y, Deng X, Jin Y, Ye P, et al. Association of frailty status with risk of fall among middle-aged and older adults in China: a nationally representative cohort study. J Nutr Health Aging. 2021;25(8):985–92. https://doi.org/10.1007/s12603-021-1655-x.
13. Global, regional, and national burden of stroke and its risk factors, 1990-2019: a systematic analysis for the global burden of disease study 2019. Lancet Neurol. 2021;20(10):795–820. https://doi.org/10.1016/s1474-4422(21)00252-0.
14. Ugur C, Gücüyener D, Uzuner N, Özkan S, Özdemir G. Characteristics of falling in patients with stroke. J Neurol Neurosurg Psychiatry. 2000;69(5):649–51. https://doi.org/10.1136/jnnp.69.5.649.
15. Batchelor FA, Mackintosh SF, Said CM, Hill KD. Falls after Stroke. Int J Stroke. 2012;7(6):482–90. https://doi.org/10.1111/j.1747-4949.2012.00796.x.
16. Indredavik B, Rohweder G, Naalsund E, Lydersen S. Medical complications in a comprehensive stroke unit and an early supported discharge service. Stroke. 2008;39(2):414–20. https://doi.org/10.1161/strokeaha.107.489294.
17. Kerse N, Parag V, Feigin VL, McNaughton H, Hackett ML, Bennett DA, et al. Falls after stroke: results from the Auckland regional community stroke (ARCOS) study, 2002 to 2003. Stroke. 2008;39(6):1890–3. https://doi.org/10.1161/strokeaha.107.509885.

18. Wong JS, Brooks D, Mansfield A. Do falls experienced during inpatient stroke rehabilitation affect length of stay, functional status, and discharge destination? Arch Phys Med Rehabil. 2016;97(4):561–6. https://doi.org/10.1016/j.apmr.2015.12.005.
19. Wei WE, De Silva DA, Chang HM, Yao J, Matchar DB, Young SHY, et al. Post-stroke patients with moderate function have the greatest risk of falls: a National Cohort Study. BMC Geriatr. 2019;19(1):373. https://doi.org/10.1186/s12877-019-1377-7.
20. Kumar A, Sidhu J, Goyal A, Tsao JW. Alzheimer Disease. In: StatPearls. Treasure Island (FL): StatPearls publishing copyright © 2023. StatPearls Publishing LLC; 2023.
21. Satış NK, Naharcı M. Predictors of two-year mortality in patients with dementia with Lewy bodies. Turk J Med Sci. 2023;53(1):366–73. https://doi.org/10.55730/1300-0144.5593.
22. Borghesani V, DeLeon J, Gorno-Tempini ML. Frontotemporal dementia: a unique window on the functional role of the temporal lobes. Handb Clin Neurol. 2022;187:429–48. https://doi.org/10.1016/b978-0-12-823493-8.00011-0.
23. Shehab A, Abdulle A. Cognitive and autonomic dysfunction measures in normal controls, white coat and borderline hypertension. BMC Cardiovasc Disord. 2011;11:3. https://doi.org/10.1186/1471-2261-11-3.
24. Lewis CE, Fine LJ, Beddhu S, Cheung AK, Cushman WC, Cutler JA, et al. Final report of a trial of intensive versus standard blood-pressure control. N Engl J Med. 2021;384(20):1921–30. https://doi.org/10.1056/NEJMoa1901281.
25. Rapp SR, Gaussoin SA, Sachs BC, Chelune G, Supiano MA, Lerner AJ, et al. Effects of intensive versus standard blood pressure control on domain-specific cognitive function: a substudy of the SPRINT randomised controlled trial. Lancet Neurol. 2020;19(11):899–907. https://doi.org/10.1016/s1474-4422(20)30319-7.
26. Scambray KA, Nguyen HL, Sajjadi SA. Association of vascular and degenerative brain pathologies and past medical history from the National Alzheimer's coordinating Center database. J Neuropathol Exp Neurol. 2023; https://doi.org/10.1093/jnen/nlad020.
27. Jin J, Wen S, Li Y, Zhou M, Duan Q, Zhou L. Factors associated with higher falling risk in elderly diabetic patients with lacunar stroke. BMC Endocr Disord. 2022;22(1):198. https://doi.org/10.1186/s12902-022-01122-3.
28. Johnstone DM, Mitrofanis J, Stone J. The brain's weakness in the face of trauma: how head trauma causes the destruction of the brain. Front Neurosci. 2023;17:1141568. https://doi.org/10.3389/fnins.2023.1141568.
29. Omalu BI, DeKosky ST, Minster RL, Kamboh MI, Hamilton RL, Wecht CH. Chronic traumatic encephalopathy in a National Football League player. Neurosurgery 2005;57(1):128–34; discussion −34. doi: https://doi.org/10.1227/01.neu.0000163407.92769.ed.
30. Xue L, Boudreau RM, Donohue JM, Zgibor JC, Marcum ZA, Costacou T, et al. Persistent polypharmacy and fall injury risk: the health, aging and body composition study. BMC Geriatr. 2021;21(1):710. https://doi.org/10.1186/s12877-021-02695-9.
31. Lee J, Negm A, Peters R, Wong EKC, Holbrook A. Deprescribing fall-risk increasing drugs (FRIDs) for the prevention of falls and fall-related complications: a systematic review and meta-analysis. BMJ Open. 2021;11(2):e035978. https://doi.org/10.1136/bmjopen-2019-035978.
32. Hart LA, Phelan EA, Yi JY, Marcum ZA, Gray SL. Use of fall risk–increasing drugs around a fall-related injury in older adults: a systematic review. J Am Geriatr Soc. 2020;68(6):1334–43. https://doi.org/10.1111/jgs.16369.
33. Virnes RE, Tiihonen M, Karttunen N, van Poelgeest EP, van der Velde N, Hartikainen S. Opioids and falls risk in older adults: a narrative review. Drugs Aging. 2022;39(3):199–207. https://doi.org/10.1007/s40266-022-00929-y.
34. Abu Bakar AA, Abdul Kadir A, Idris NS, Mohd Nawi SN. Older adults with hypertension: prevalence of falls and their associated factors. Int J Environ Res Public Health. 2021;18(16) https://doi.org/10.3390/ijerph18168257.
35. Albasri A, Hattle M, Koshiaris C, Dunnigan A, Paxton B, Fox SE, et al. Association between antihypertensive treatment and adverse events: systematic review and meta-analysis. BMJ. 2021;372:n189. https://doi.org/10.1136/bmj.n189.

36. Anderson TS, Jing B, Auerbach A, Wray CM, Lee S, Boscardin WJ, et al. Clinical outcomes after intensifying antihypertensive medication regimens among older adults at hospital discharge. JAMA Intern Med. 2019;179(11):1528–36. https://doi.org/10.1001/jamainternmed.2019.3007.
37. Tinetti ME, Han L, Lee DSH, McAvay GJ, Peduzzi P, Gross CP, et al. Antihypertensive medications and serious fall injuries in a nationally representative sample of older adults. JAMA Intern Med. 2014;174(4):588–95. https://doi.org/10.1001/jamainternmed.2013.14764.
38. Yang Y, Hu X, Zhang Q, Zou R. Diabetes mellitus and risk of falls in older adults: a systematic review and meta-analysis. Age Ageing. 2016;45(6):761–7. https://doi.org/10.1093/ageing/afw140.
39. Bergenstal RM, Beck RW, Close KL, Grunberger G, Sacks DB, Kowalski A, et al. Glucose management indicator (GMI): a new term for estimating A1C from continuous glucose monitoring. Diabetes Care. 2018;41(11):2275–80. https://doi.org/10.2337/dc18-1581.
40. KDIGO. 2020 clinical practice guideline for diabetes Management in Chronic Kidney Disease. Kidney Int. 2020;98(4s):S1–s115. https://doi.org/10.1016/j.kint.2020.06.019.
41. Fonseca V, Kohzuma T, Galindo RJ, DeSouza C. KDIGO recommendations for the evaluation of glycemic control in advanced chronic kidney disease. Kidney Int. 2022;101(2):420. https://doi.org/10.1016/j.kint.2021.11.020.
42. Isshiki K, Nishio T, Isono M, Makiishi T, Shikano T, Tomita K, et al. Glycated albumin predicts the risk of mortality in type 2 diabetic patients on hemodialysis: evaluation of a target level for improving survival. Ther Apher Dial. 2014;18(5):434–42. https://doi.org/10.1111/1744-9987.12123.
43. Galindo RJ, Beck RW, Scioscia MF, Umpierrez GE, Tuttle KR. Glycemic monitoring and management in advanced chronic kidney disease. Endocr Rev. 2020;41(5):756–74. https://doi.org/10.1210/endrev/bnaa017.
44. Battistella M, Ng P. Addressing polypharmacy in outpatient dialysis units. Clin J Am Soc Nephrol. 2021;16(1):144. https://doi.org/10.2215/CJN.05270420.
45. Quesada V, Freitas-Rodríguez S, Miller J, Pérez-Silva JG, Jiang Z-F, Tapia W, et al. Giant tortoise genomes provide insights into longevity and age-related disease. Nat Ecol Evol. 2019;3(1):87–95. https://doi.org/10.1038/s41559-018-0733-x.
46. Chang JT, Ganz DA. Quality indicators for falls and mobility problems in vulnerable elders. J Am Geriatr Soc. 2007;55(Suppl 2):S327–34. https://doi.org/10.1111/j.1532-5415.2007.01339.x.
47. Fuller GF. Falls in the elderly. Am Fam Physician. 2000;61(7):2159–68, 73–4
48. Moreland B, Kakara R, Henry A. Trends in nonfatal falls and fall-related injuries among adults aged ≥65 years - United States, 2012-2018. MMWR Morb Mortal Wkly Rep. 2020;69(27):875–81. https://doi.org/10.15585/mmwr.mm6927a5.
49. Shen Y. Role of nutritional vitamin D in chronic kidney disease-mineral and bone disorder: a narrative review. Medicine (Baltimore). 2023;102(14):e33477. https://doi.org/10.1097/md.0000000000033477.
50. Angalakuditi MV, Gomes J, Coley KC. Impact of drug use and comorbidities on in-hospital falls in patients with chronic kidney disease. Ann Pharmacother. 2007;41(10):1638–43. https://doi.org/10.1345/aph.1H631.
51. Kutner NG, Zhang R, Huang Y, Wasse H. Falls among hemodialysis patients: potential opportunities for prevention? Clin Kidney J. 2014;7(3):257–63. https://doi.org/10.1093/ckj/sfu034.
52. Danese MD, Kim J, Doan QV, Dylan M, Griffiths R, Chertow GM. PTH and the risks for hip, vertebral, and pelvic fractures among patients on dialysis. Am J Kidney Dis. 2006;47(1):149–56. https://doi.org/10.1053/j.ajkd.2005.09.024.
53. Cohen-Solal M, Funck-Brentano T, Ureña TP. Bone fragility in patients with chronic kidney disease. Endocr Connect. 2020;9(4):R93–r101. https://doi.org/10.1530/ec-20-0039.
54. Hansen D, Olesen JB, Gislason GH, Abrahamsen B, Hommel K. Risk of fracture in adults on renal replacement therapy: a Danish national cohort study. Nephrology Dialysis Transplantation. 2016;31(10):1654–62. https://doi.org/10.1093/ndt/gfw073.

55. Xu Q, Ou X, Li J. The risk of falls among the aging population: a systematic review and meta-analysis. Front Public Health. 2022;10:902599. https://doi.org/10.3389/fpubh.2022.902599.
56. Song Y, Deng Y, Li J, Hao B, Cai Y, Chen J, et al. Associations of falls and severe falls with blood pressure and frailty among Chinese community-dwelling oldest olds: the Chinese longitudinal health and longevity study. Aging (Albany N Y). 2021;13(12):16527–40. https://doi.org/10.18632/aging.203174.
57. Bromfield SG, Ngameni CA, Colantonio LD, Bowling CB, Shimbo D, Reynolds K, et al. Blood pressure, antihypertensive polypharmacy, frailty, and risk for serious fall injuries among older treated adults with hypertension. Hypertension. 2017;70(2):259–66. https://doi.org/10.1161/hypertensionaha.116.09390.
58. Karamanou M, Protogerou A, Tsoucalas G, Androutsos G, Poulakou-Rebelakou E. Milestones in the history of diabetes mellitus: the main contributors. World J Diabetes. 2016;7(1):1–7. https://doi.org/10.4239/wjd.v7.i1.1.
59. Napoli N, Chandran M, Pierroz DD, Abrahamsen B, Schwartz AV, Ferrari SL. Mechanisms of diabetes mellitus-induced bone fragility. Nat Rev Endocrinol. 2017;13(4):208–19. https://doi.org/10.1038/nrendo.2016.153.
60. Zhao Q, Khedkar SV, Johnson KC. Weight loss interventions and skeletal health in persons with diabetes. Curr Osteoporos Rep. 2022;20(5):240–8. https://doi.org/10.1007/s11914-022-00744-9.
61. Nomoto H. Fixed-ratio combinations of basal insulin and glucagon-like peptide-1 receptor agonists as a promising strategy for treating diabetes. World J Diabetes. 2023;14(3):188–97. https://doi.org/10.4239/wjd.v14.i3.188.
62. Shi Q, Nong K, Vandvik PO, Guyatt GH, Schnell O, Rydén L, et al. Benefits and harms of drug treatment for type 2 diabetes: systematic review and network meta-analysis of randomised controlled trials. BMJ. 2023;381:e074068. https://doi.org/10.1136/bmj-2022-074068.
63. Volgman AS, Nair G, Lyubarova R, Merchant FM, Mason P, Curtis AB, et al. Management of Atrial Fibrillation in patients 75 years and older: JACC state-of-the-art review. J Am Coll Cardiol. 2022;79(2):166–79. https://doi.org/10.1016/j.jacc.2021.10.037.
64. Holmqvist F, Hellkamp AS, Lee KL, Lamas GA, Daubert JP. Adverse effects of first-degree AV-block in patients with sinus node dysfunction: data from the mode selection trial. Pacing Clin Electrophysiol. 2014;37(9):1111–9. https://doi.org/10.1111/pace.12404.
65. Crisel RK, Farzaneh-Far R, Na B, Whooley MA. First-degree atrioventricular block is associated with heart failure and death in persons with stable coronary artery disease: data from the heart and soul study. Eur Heart J. 2011;32(15):1875–80. https://doi.org/10.1093/eurheartj/ehr139.
66. Rosenblatt AG, Ayers CR, Rao A, Howell SJ, Hendren NS, Zadikany RH, et al. New-onset atrial fibrillation in patients hospitalized with COVID-19: results from the American Heart Association COVID-19 cardiovascular registry. Circ Arrhythm Electrophysiol. 2022;15(5):e010666. https://doi.org/10.1161/CIRCEP.121.010666.
67. Dallmeier D, Klenk J, Peter RS, Denkinger M, Peter R, Rapp K, et al. A prospective assessment of cardiac biomarkers for hemodynamic stress and necrosis and the risk of falls among older people: the ActiFE study. Eur J Epidemiol. 2016;31(4):427–35. https://doi.org/10.1007/s10654-015-0059-9.
68. Oliveira CC, Annoni R, Lee AL, McGinley J, Irving LB, Denehy L. Falls prevalence and risk factors in people with chronic obstructive pulmonary disease: a systematic review. Respir Med. 2021;176:106284. https://doi.org/10.1016/j.rmed.2020.106284.
69. Yentes JM, Liu WY, Zhang K, Markvicka E, Rennard SI. Updated perspectives on the role of biomechanics in COPD: considerations for the clinician. Int J Chron Obstruct Pulmon Dis. 2022;17:2653–75. https://doi.org/10.2147/copd.S339195.
70. Zhang Y, Cifuentes M, Gao X, Amaral G, Tucker KL. Age- and gender-specific associations between insomnia and falls in Boston Puerto Rican adults. Qual Life Res. 2017;26(1):25–34. https://doi.org/10.1007/s11136-016-1374-7.

71. Hayley AC, Williams LJ, Kennedy GA, Holloway KL, Berk M, Brennan-Olsen SL, et al. Excessive daytime sleepiness and falls among older men and women: cross-sectional examination of a population-based sample. BMC Geriatr. 2015;15(1):74. https://doi.org/10.1186/s12877-015-0068-2.
72. Roepke SK, Ancoli-Israel S. Sleep disorders in the elderly. Indian J Med Res. 2010;131:302–10.
73. Tinetti ME, Williams TF, Mayewski R. Fall risk index for elderly patients based on number of chronic disabilities. Am J Med. 1986;80(3):429–34. https://doi.org/10.1016/0002-9343(86)90717-5.
74. Fadem SZ. One year later. Perit Dial Int. 1999;19(6):509–11.
75. Campbell G, Wolfe RA, Klem ML. Risk factors for falls in adult cancer survivors: an integrative review. Rehabil Nurs. 2018;43(4):201–13. https://doi.org/10.1097/rnj.0000000000000173.
76. Doré AL, Golightly YM, Mercer VS, Shi XA, Renner JB, Jordan JM, et al. Lower-extremity osteoarthritis and the risk of falls in a community-based longitudinal study of adults with and without osteoarthritis. Arthritis Care Res (Hoboken). 2015;67(5):633–9. https://doi.org/10.1002/acr.22499.
77. Bu F, Abell J, Zaninotto P, Fancourt D. A longitudinal analysis of loneliness, social isolation and falls amongst older people in England. Sci Rep. 2020;10(1):20064. https://doi.org/10.1038/s41598-020-77104-z.
78. Shuyi O, Zheng C, Lin Z, Zhang X, Li H, Fang Y, et al. Risk factors of falls in elderly patients with visual impairment. Front Public Health. 2022;10:984199. https://doi.org/10.3389/fpubh.2022.984199.
79. Mehta J, Czanner G, Harding S, Newsham D, Robinson J. Visual risk factors for falls in older adults: a case-control study. BMC Geriatr. 2022;22(1):134. https://doi.org/10.1186/s12877-022-02784-3.
80. Ghahramani M, Stirling D, Naghdy F, Naghdy G, Potter J. Body postural sway analysis in older people with different fall histories. Med Biol Eng Comput. 2019;57(2):533–42. https://doi.org/10.1007/s11517-018-1901-5.
81. Verghese J, LeValley A, Hall CB, Katz MJ, Ambrose AF, Lipton RB. Epidemiology of gait disorders in community-residing older adults. J Am Geriatr Soc. 2006;54(2):255–61. https://doi.org/10.1111/j.1532-5415.2005.00580.x.
82. Verghese J, Ambrose AF, Lipton RB, Wang C. Neurological gait abnormalities and risk of falls in older adults. J Neurol. 2010;257(3):392–8. https://doi.org/10.1007/s00415-009-5332-y.
83. Craig JJ, Bruetsch AP, Huisinga JM. Coordination of trunk and foot acceleration during gait is affected by walking velocity and fall history in elderly adults. Aging Clin Exp Res. 2019;31(7):943–50. https://doi.org/10.1007/s40520-018-1036-4.
84. Thaler-Kall K, Peters A, Thorand B, Grill E, Autenrieth CS, Horsch A, et al. Description of spatio-temporal gait parameters in elderly people and their association with history of falls: results of the population-based cross-sectional KORA-age study. BMC Geriatr. 2015;15(1):32. https://doi.org/10.1186/s12877-015-0032-1.
85. Rajan V, Mitch WE. Ubiquitin, proteasomes and proteolytic mechanisms activated by kidney disease. Biochim Biophys Acta. 2008;1782(12):795–9. https://doi.org/10.1016/j.bbadis.2008.07.007.
86. Reid MB. Response of the ubiquitin-proteasome pathway to changes in muscle activity. Am J Physiol Regul Integr Comp Physiol. 2005;288(6):R1423–31. https://doi.org/10.1152/ajpregu.00545.2004.
87. Yeung SSY, Reijnierse EM, Pham VK, Trappenburg MC, Lim WK, Meskers CGM, et al. Sarcopenia and its association with falls and fractures in older adults: a systematic review and meta-analysis. J Cachexia Sarcopenia Muscle. 2019;10(3):485–500. https://doi.org/10.1002/jcsm.12411.
88. Tembo MC, Mohebbi M, Holloway-Kew KL, Gaston J, Sui SX, Brennan-Olsen SL, et al. The contribution of musculoskeletal factors to physical frailty: a cross-sectional study. BMC Musculoskelet Disord. 2021;22(1):921. https://doi.org/10.1186/s12891-021-04795-4.

89. Rath B, Nam J, Knobloch TJ, Lannutti JJ, Agarwal S. Compressive forces induce osteogenic gene expression in calvarial osteoblasts. J Biomech. 2008;41(5):1095–103. https://doi.org/10.1016/j.jbiomech.2007.11.024.
90. Wang D, Wang H, Gao F, Wang K, Dong F. ClC-3 promotes osteogenic differentiation in MC3T3-E1 cell after dynamic compression. J Cell Biochem. 2017;118(6):1606–13. https://doi.org/10.1002/jcb.25823.
91. Xia W, Cooper C, Li M, Xu L, Rizzoli R, Zhu M, et al. East meets west: current practices and policies in the management of musculoskeletal aging. Aging Clin Exp Res. 2019;31(10):1351–73. https://doi.org/10.1007/s40520-019-01282-8.
92. Metcalfe D. The pathophysiology of osteoporotic hip fracture. McGill J Med. 2008;11(1):51–7.
93. Florencio-Silva R, Sasso GR, Sasso-Cerri E, Simões MJ, Cerri PS. Biology of bone tissue: structure, function, and factors that influence bone cells. Biomed Res Int. 2015;2015:421746. https://doi.org/10.1155/2015/421746.
94. Aquino-Martínez R, Artigas N, Gámez B, Rosa JL, Ventura F. Extracellular calcium promotes bone formation from bone marrow mesenchymal stem cells by amplifying the effects of BMP-2 on SMAD signalling. PLoS One. 2017;12(5):e0178158. https://doi.org/10.1371/journal.pone.0178158.
95. Holvik K, Ellingsen CL, Solbakken SM, Finnes TE, Talsnes O, Grimnes G, et al. Cause-specific excess mortality after hip fracture: the Norwegian epidemiologic osteoporosis studies (NOREPOS). BMC Geriatr. 2023;23(1):201. https://doi.org/10.1186/s12877-023-03910-5.
96. Hamrick I, Norton D, Birstler J, Chen G, Cruz L, Hanrahan L. Association between dehydration and falls. Mayo Clin Proc Innov Qual Outcomes. 2020;4(3):259–65. https://doi.org/10.1016/j.mayocpiqo.2020.01.003.
97. Canaud B, Kooman JP, Selby NM, Taal MW, Francis S, Maierhofer A, et al. Dialysis-induced cardiovascular and multiorgan morbidity. Kidney Int Rep. 2020;5(11):1856–69. https://doi.org/10.1016/j.ekir.2020.08.031.
98. Roberts RG, Kenny RA, Brierley EJ. Are elderly haemodialysis patients at risk of falls and postural hypotension? Int Urol Nephrol. 2003;35(3):415–21. https://doi.org/10.1023/b:urol.0000022866.07751.4a.

Chapter 3
Mechanical Falls

3.1 Introduction

Mechanical falls occur due to external factors in contrast to intrinsic medical disorders. These factors are generally environmental but often occur in combination with a medical condition. Many environmental falls are preventable, but it takes education, awareness, and implementing strategies that involve a community to change to a culture of safety that can focus on fall prevention.

This is a worthwhile aim. The National Safety Council reports that an older adult dies of a fall every 20 mins (**https://www.nsc.org/community-safety/safety-topics/older-adult-falls**). In a global review of the medical literature, efforts to make the home environment safer led to a 26% reduction in the rate of falls. In those with a higher risk of falling, the reduction rate was 38% [1].

Environmental fall hazards are associated with obstacles blocking access to the toilet, shower, or tub, poor or absent lighting, and slippery or uneven flooring, with most falls occurring in the bathroom. The risk of an environmental fall increases with age. Falls decrease when slick flooring is addressed, grab bars and handrails are installed, and night-lights are used. Avoiding clutter on the floor and using grabbers rather than ladders to access difficult-to-access objects also reduce falls. Ensuring adequate room for maneuverability and arranging furniture to avoid trip hazards are also helpful [2].

3.2 What Is Balance?

Mechanical falls can occur because of a sudden loss of balance. Balance happens when the brain integrates sensory information from the surface one is walking on (called proprioception) from the inner ear and the eyes.

3.2.1 Inner Ear (See Fig. 3.1)

The ear not only senses sound but also balance. The sound activates the eardrum or tympanic membrane through vibrations sensed by three tiny bones in the inner ear (Fig. 3.1). The sound waves into the spiral-shaped cochlea, where they vibrate a gel moving sensitive hairlike structures that convert the waves and vibrations to nerve impulses that are sent along the cochlear nerve to the brain.

The inner ear is like a gyroscope. It evolved millions of years ago from primitive sensing mechanisms—even jellyfish, primitive insect ancestors, clams, snails, and starfish have sensory organs called statocysts that can detect changes in gravity and acceleration. These primitive animals could use nerve impulses to sense water currents and determine the best opportunities for food. These structures evolved into an inner ear with three semicircular canals filled with fluid and lined with hair cells that determine position and acceleration. As our heads move, the fluid shifts move the hair cells that trigger signals. These signals travel along the vestibular nerve to the brain, where they register balance. The balance system in the brain also receives signals from the eyes.

Balance disorders are associated with aging and chronic diseases. In many people, they may not be noticeable until trying to stand on one leg. However, even the slightest decrease in balance ability can lead to a mechanical fall if the environment is unsafe.

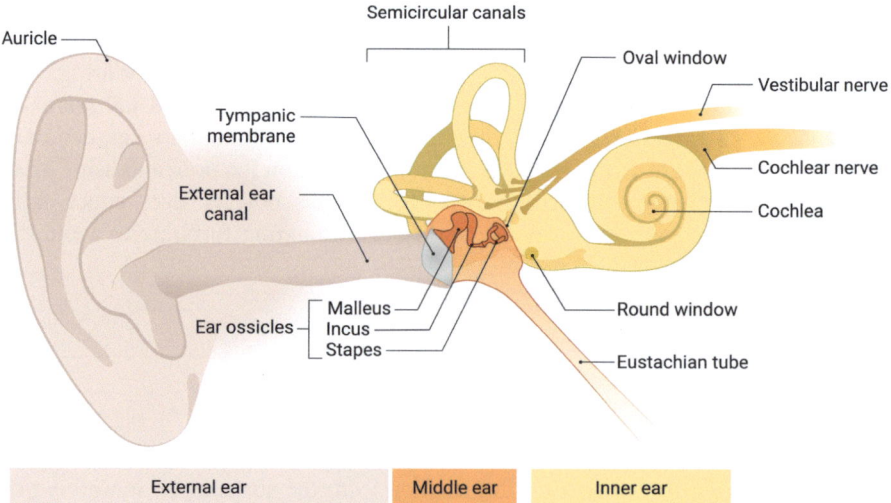

Fig. 3.1 Anatomy of the ear. (Created with BioRender.com)

3.2.2 Eyesight

The eyes are important balance tools because they can sense our position in relation to our environment. Around 20% of the nerves in the eye interact with the balance system in the brain.

3.2.3 Proprioception or Sense of Position

Our joints, muscle, and feet are all interconnected to a system that travels through the spinal cord and offers feedback to the brain regarding our position. The brain integrates the signals from peripheral receptors and then adjusts our posture to maintain balance. Proprioception is the term used to describe how we sense position; it is also called kinesthesia. It allows us to seamlessly judge limb and body positions and is tied not just to the sensation but the control of movement even when the eyes are closed.

3.2.4 Body Sway

Normally we sway slightly when standing. This is because the body constantly integrates sensations from our eyes, inner ear, and peripheral receptors. Swaying can be exaggerated in persons who are older. There are measurable differences in body sway between those who are at risk of falling [3].

3.2.5 Being Off-Balance

Disrupting either proprioception, vision, or the inner ear function results in compensation by the other two. However, when two of the three systems, the inner ear, proprioception, and eyesight, are impaired, we tend to lose balance and fall. This is especially true in the elderly or those with chronic illnesses, for their balance is already compromised.

3.3 Mechanical (Environmental) Reasons for Falls

Table 3.1 highlights how people can fall at home, outdoors, participating in recreational events, or when working or traveling. There is considerable overlap, and this list is far from complete.

Table 3.1 Common ways and places to fall. Note the overlap

Home
1 Not using the handrails on stairs
2 Slippery floors and surfaces
3 Bathrooms—mats and grab bars
4 Uneven surfaces (jutting surfaces and small steps)
5 Slips—wrinkled carpet
6 Ladder accidents
7 Tripping over clutter
8 Not using the night-light
9 Not using a walker, cane, or assistive device
10 Wheelchair safety
11 Standing too quickly
Outdoors
1 Hiking without sticks
2 Improper footwear
3 Not wearing a hat
4 Not wearing sunscreen
5 Inadequate water supply
6 Not using a headlamp in darkness
7 Dangerous rocks and edges—no support
8 Lack of guardrail safety

3.4 Home

3.4.1 Not Using the Handrails on Stairs

On July 14, 2022, Ivana Trump was found dead near the bottom of the spiral staircase in her luxurious Upper East Side residence. Neighbors had noticed that her health and posture had been declining and that she was walking with a cane. The Chief Medical Examiner for New York ruled the death the result of blunt impact trauma to the torso. Falls and injuries related to stairs are common. In a review of emergency room visits, there were 24,760,843 stair-related injuries over a 23-year period. This averaged to just over one million stair injuries a year. The majority (67.2%) were either children under 11 years old or persons over 60. Fractures occurred in 19.3% of persons. Most injuries were to the lower extremities, but 21.6% were to the head and neck [4].

Falling on the stairs is the second most common cause of injury in persons over age 65. Falls downstairs are common causes of foot or ankle fractures and shoulder injuries. The risk of a fracture to the ankle or foot from a staircase accident is twice that of one standing still [5]. Falls downstairs occur most commonly because one loses balance. Those with poor postural control, gait instability, or compromised ability to regulate body sway are likely to have difficulty negotiating stairs [6]. Postural control is worsened with osteoarthritis and knee instability [7]. Ms. Trump's unfortunate death highlights that those with age-related complications must exert extra vigilance when climbing or descending stairs.

3.4 Home

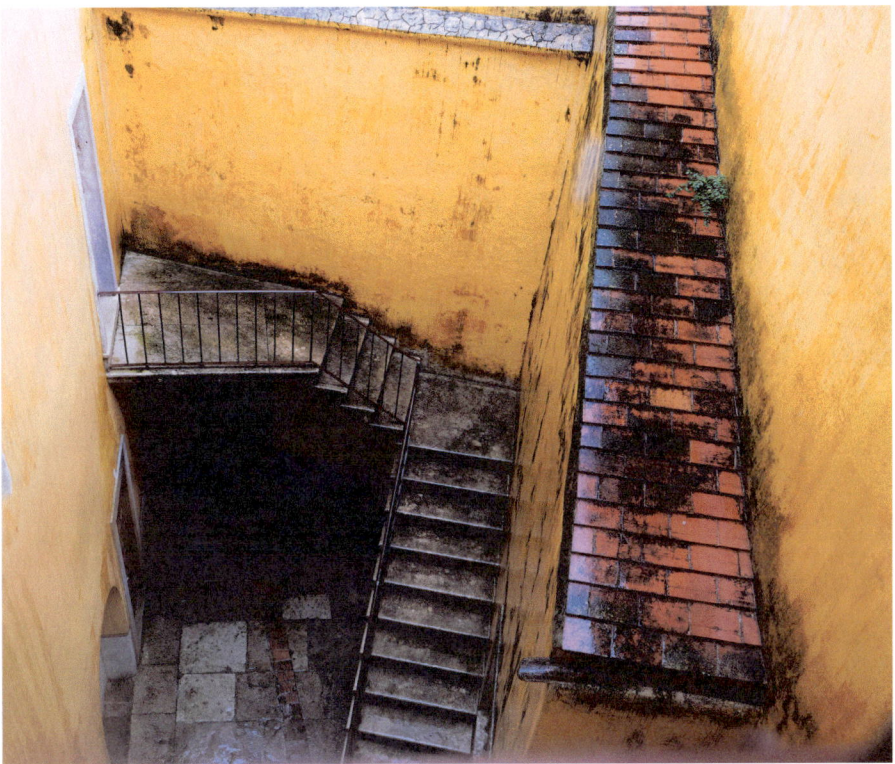

Fig. 3.2 Handrails prevent falls. Trying to walk on the stairs while holding objects and not holding on to the rails is a fall risk, particularly in the elderly

Those with even minor balance difficulties should exercise caution, wear proper soles with ample traction, hold the handrail at all times when ascending or descending stairs, and only climb stairs when the lighting is adequate (see Fig. 3.2).

3.4.2 Slippery Floors and Surfaces

Floor surfaces account for a majority of fall injuries. If a floor is slippery for any reason, it can present a fall hazard. Ideally, a home, apartment, clinic, or retail establishment will have flooring that will not pose a risk for a person to slip and fall. While ceramic tile is often used for flooring, there is considerable variation in surface friction. Surfaces with low slip resistance do not allow pedestrian footwear to grip the floor. Many surfaces in buildings do not allow safe movement of people, especially when wet. This is also true on staircases. In general, surfaces that are clean and dry pose less slip risk. Dust on the floor acts like ball bearings and creates a slick surface.

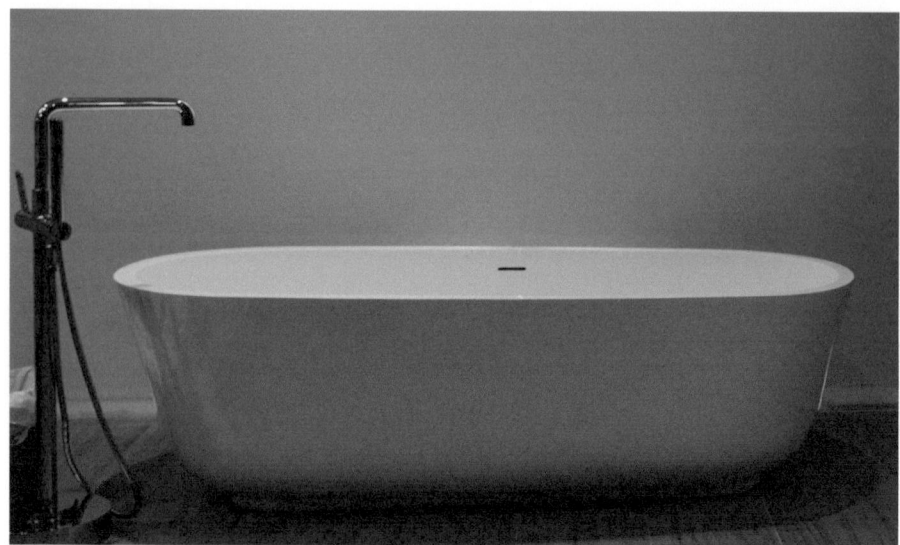

Fig. 3.3 Falling in the bathtub is the most common cause of death from falls

It is important to follow the manufacturer's instructions when cleaning a floor. Overcleaning may remove a protective surface. A floor that is improperly cleaned may either be over-waxed and slick, or alternately, spilled food and liquids may be left on the floor. Highly polished surfaces that are safe when dry can become slippery if wet.

The coefficient of friction (COF) or resistance that determines slip potential depends upon the type of finish [8]. The COF is published by the tile manufacturer, as is the newer dynamic COF (DCOF). A zero COF rating is very slippery, and a slick tile may be rated as low as 0.04. Floors with a DCOF rating of less than 0.42 are a slip hazard when wet. Honed natural stone is slippery like glass. Terracotta and quarry tile have high COF ratings, as does brick.

Improper footwear and either water or oil spilled on a slick floor may be treacherous for one who is prone to fall. The Tile Council of North America (**https://tcnatile.com/**) had developed industry criteria and performs COF and other tests like the dynamic coefficient of friction (DCOF). Standards have been developed and published for various establishments. External floor and poor decks must have a DCOF of ≥ 0.60 when wet, and ramps, stairs, wheelchair ramps, and pedestrian sidewalks must have a DCOF of ≥ 0.65.

3.4.3 Bathrooms: Mats and Grab Bars

Falling backward from a standing position while getting out of the bathtub is the main cause of death from falls (see Fig. 3.3). It is probably associated with a drop in blood pressure while bathing in hot water. In a Japanese study, 90% of the deaths occurred in persons ≥ 65 years old and in the winter when there was the greatest

3.4 Home

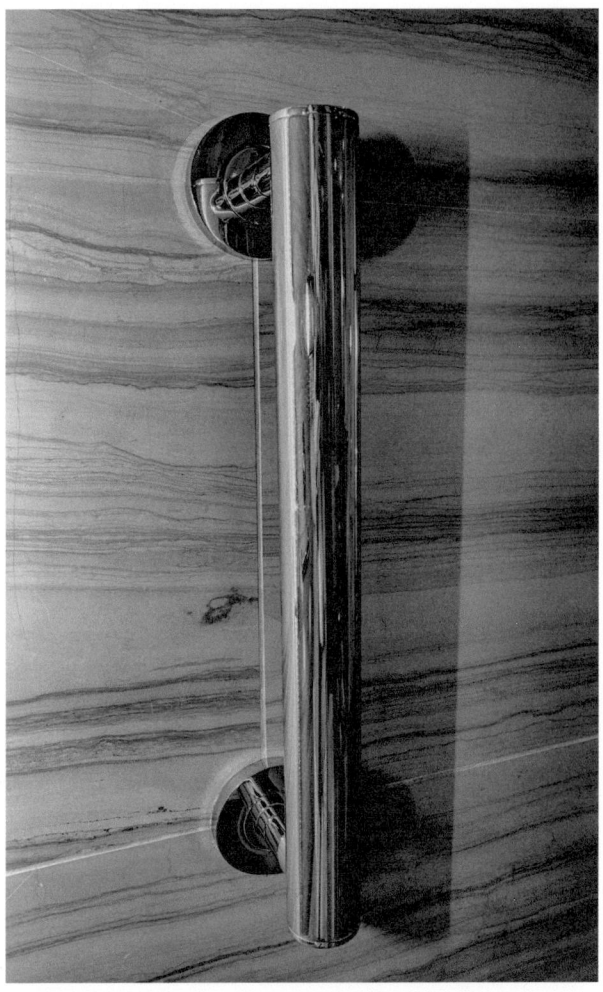

Fig. 3.4 The loss of balance is a major reason for falling. Using a grab bar can prevent a serious injury

difference between environmental temperature and that of the water [9, 10]. Less than half of the homes in the USA have handrails or grab bars in the bathroom. In a telephone survey of homes, the families with at least one person with a disability, only 40.4% had installed grab bars or handrails in the bathtub or shower, and only 71% had mats or nonskid strips in the tub or shower [11]. In Canada, only 34.6% of households have grab bars (see Fig. 3.4) [12].

Grab bars come in various configurations. It was found that with the sudden loss of balance while bathing, 59.4% of older adults use the grab bars to regain balance as compared to 13.6% of their younger counterparts. Vertical bars on a side wall are favored [13]. Grab bars should be installed to create the safest possible condition when getting in or out of the tub or shower and when controlling it. The Americans with Disabilities Act (ADA) website published guidelines and standards that cover this safety concern (**https://www.ada.gov/law-and-regs/design-standards/standards-guidance/**).

3.4.4 Uneven Surfaces (Jutting Surfaces and Small Steps)

Falls can occur on uneven or jutting surfaces. Uneven surfaces can develop indoors because of worn or frayed spots on carpeting, chipped tiles, or loose flooring. When outdoors, gravel, snow, ice, leaves, and uneven pavement cause 19 times as many serious injuries as collision road accidents [14] (see Fig. 3.5). It has been reported

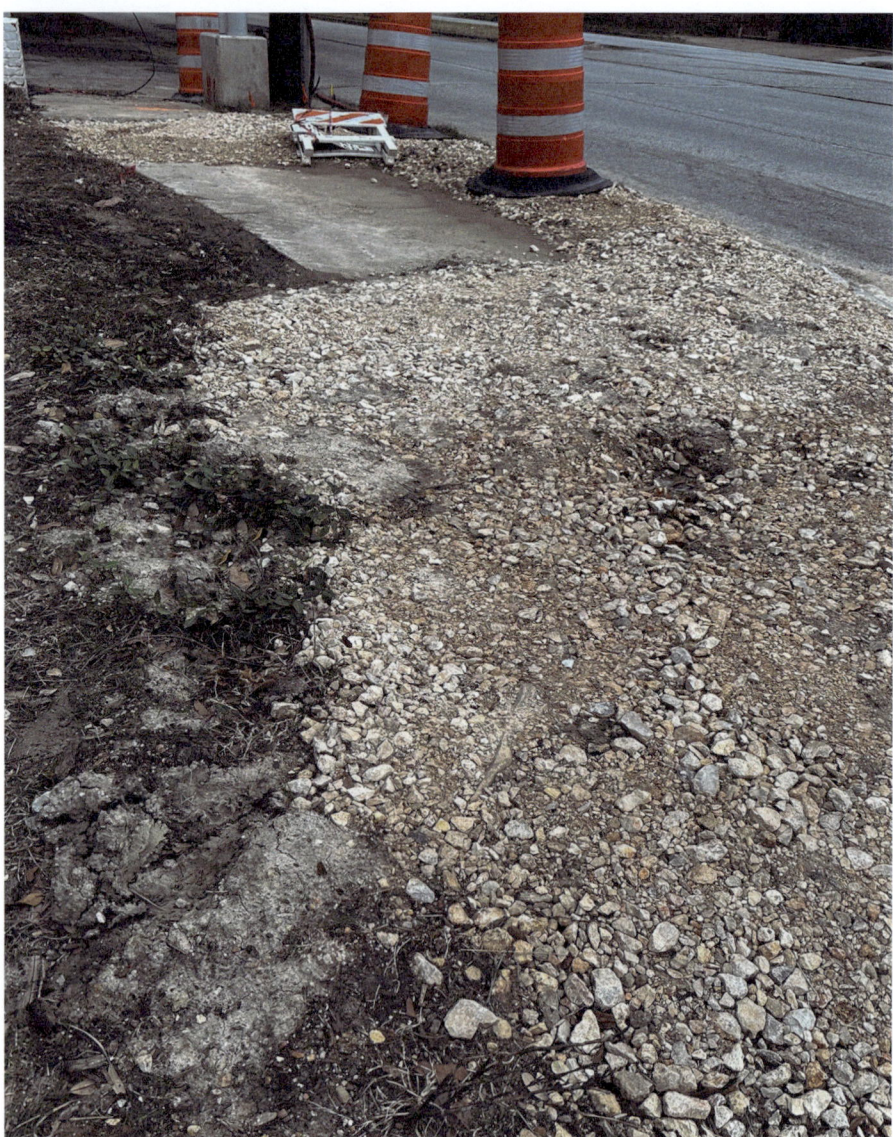

Fig. 3.5 It is easy to trip over an uneven surface. Those with impairments should use caution

that 12% of all road fatalities and serious injuries occur in pedestrians while walking. The most common injury from a fall while walking is a fracture [15]. The anatomy of an accident related to an uneven surface or flooring that is not clean, dry, and level or otherwise unsafe. An individual with an impaired sense of balance/gait disorder or is distracted and inattentive to the potential disaster on the floor or road cannot maintain a stable gait. Most commonly, it is a combination of poor balance and inattentiveness that leads to a loss of footing. The person cannot regain stability but is carried forward by momentum and falls either on an outstretched hand sustaining a wrist fracture or falls directly onto a hip, sustaining a fractured femur, or sprains or fractures an ankle. Many other factors play a role in an accident happening—poor lighting, improper footwear, and patient deconditioning are also factors.

Jutting objects (see Fig. 3.6) especially tree branches and cabinet doors that have been left open are hazards because a person can accidentally hit their head against them. Potential injuries include trauma to the eye or face, a concussion, or even significant brain injury. Jutting objects also are a fall risk.

3.4.5 Slips: Wrinkled Rugs

Rugs and carpets are both floor coverings (see Fig. 3.7). Carpets generally are fixed to a floor and cover a larger space. Rugs are easily moved. If carpets or rugs are not secured, they can easily slip and move when walked on. This can throw one off-balance, resulting in a fall. A carpet with an uneven, wrinkled surface creates a trip hazard. Carpet that is damaged and worn can also become a trip hazard. In one study of carpeting accidents, there were nearly 38,000 injuries in persons ≥ 65 years old. Carpeting accounts for 54.2% of injuries, and rugs 45.8%. Most falls occur at home, and 35.7% occur in the bathroom. The common scenario is hurrying to the bathroom and slipping on a wet transition from one type of surface (i.e., rug) to another (i.e., a hard tile floor). Among those injured, 10,016 had a concussion, and 15,861 had a fracture [16].

3.4.6 Ladder Accidents

Ladder accidents are very dangerous and can cause fatal falls in the elderly (see Fig. 3.8). As we age, we sometimes forget our present capabilities but recall when we could effortlessly ascend ladders. Balance losses can be subtle, and what was easy in the past may become a present threat. With impaired balance, it is often best to rely on a friend, loved one, or neighbor to grab the out-of-reach box or change the light bulb. Accidents occur when one does not hold on or loses footing. Ladders that are set up incorrectly account for around 40% of accidents. Another reason for accidents is using a ladder that is not the correct size, forcing one to attempt to ascend to the top step. Many weekend fix-it-yourself homeowners use ladders improperly, having no realization of their potential danger, and can borrow tips from the National

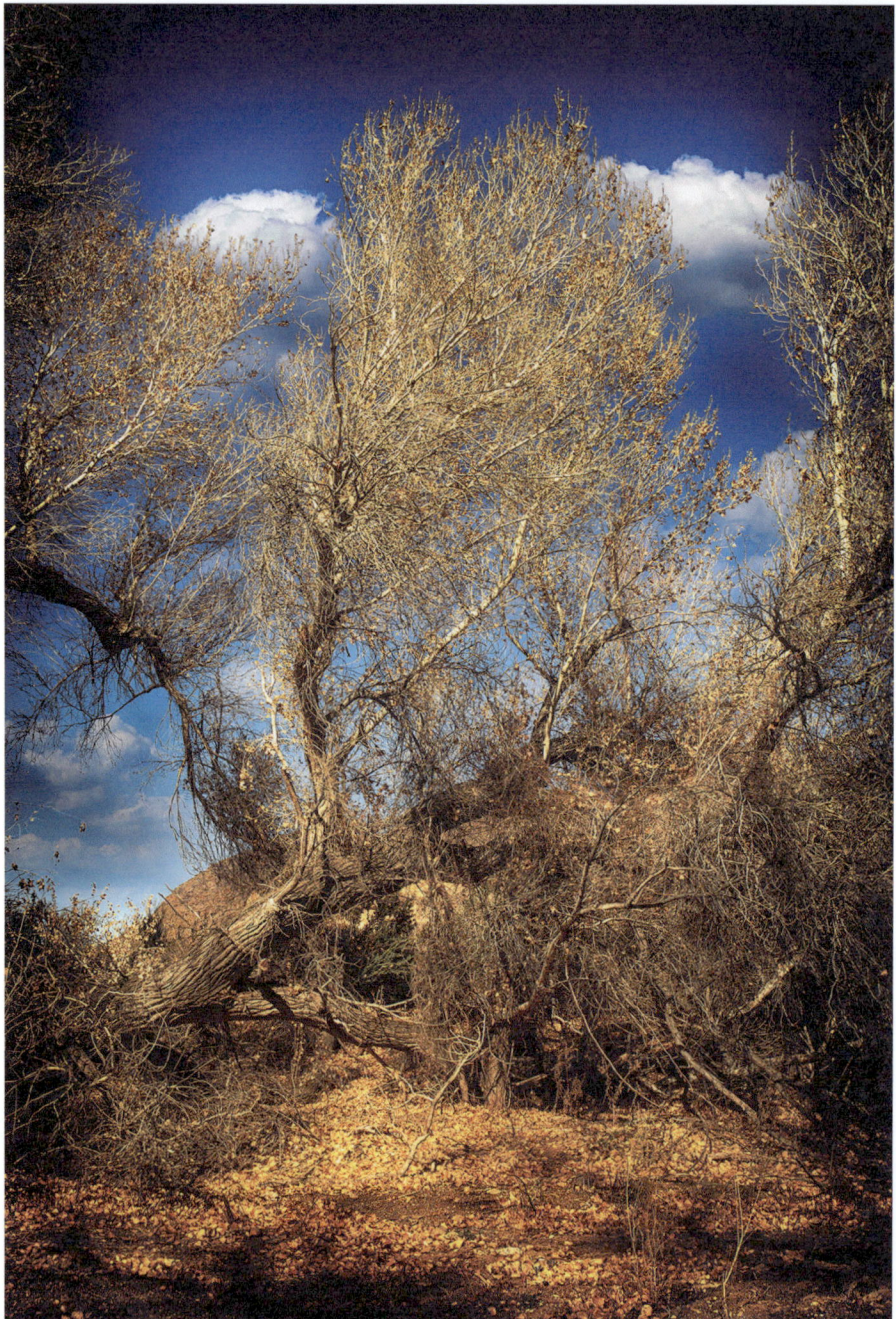

Fig. 3.6 Jutting objects like fallen trees on the trail can cause substantial injuries. Open cabinet doors can also cause head trauma

3.4 Home

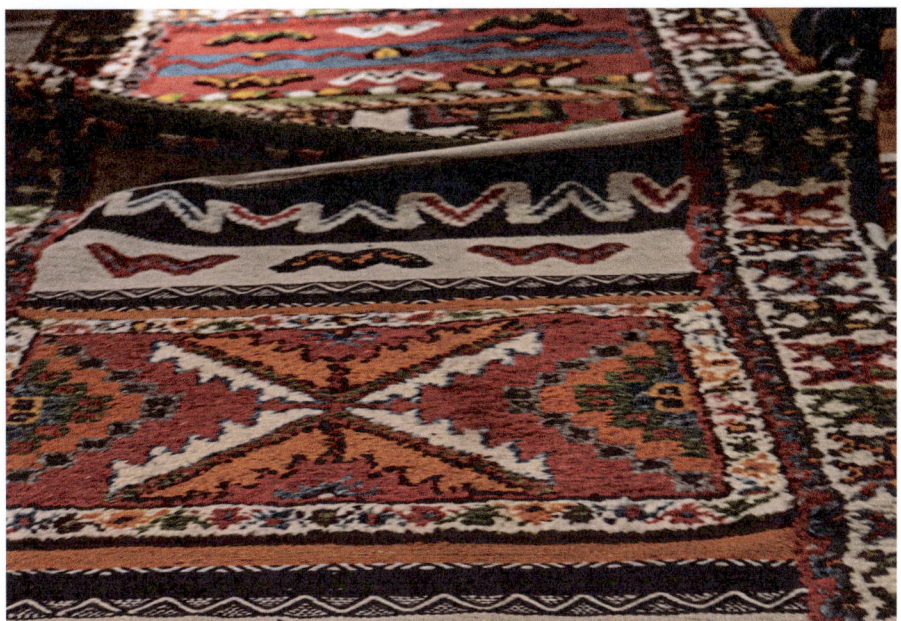

Fig. 3.7 While often beautiful and expensive, a poorly secured rug can lead to a dangerous fall

Institute for Occupational Safety and Health (NIOSH) regarding ladder safety (**https://www.cdc.gov/niosh/newsroom/feature/ladder-safety.html**).

Falls can often be avoided by using a hand extension reacher grabber to extend one's reach. It is ergonomic, slim, and lightweight and has a powerful grip. The reacher grabber reduces the risk of falling and can decrease movements that lead to strains, allowing those who have limited mobility or who are a fall risk to remain independent (Fig. 3.9).

3.4.7 Tripping over Clutter

While some falls are related to slipping on a slick floor, around half are related to tripping over cluttered obstacles that have been left on the floor, especially in those who are elderly and have gait or balance disturbances (Fig. 3.10). Tripping occurs when one's foot suddenly and unexpectedly comes into contact with an obstacle that was not cleared with walking. Tripping is set up by the swinging of the foot. Footwear, walking speed, and object visibility can make a difference in the risk. Also, in darkness, vision cannot contribute to balance control. Lighting and depth perception can help reduce falls. Risk factors also include wires and cords that are strung across the floor. Improperly placed furniture can also be a source of a fall, as can dim lighting. Night-lights are more effective when placed in the front rather

Fig. 3.8 Ladders at either home or the workplace should be set up appropriately to avoid malfunction and secondary injury

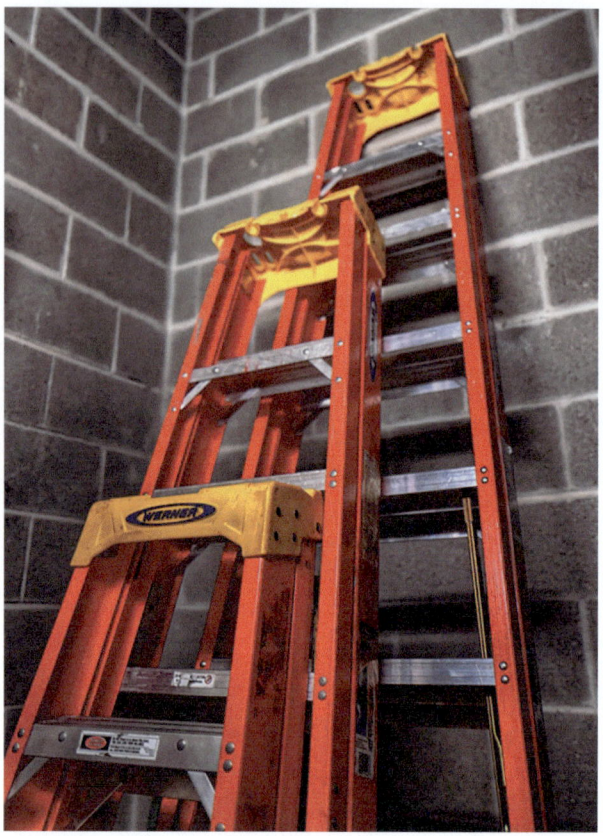

Fig. 3.9 Reacher grabbers are inexpensive and useful for getting objects that are out of reach

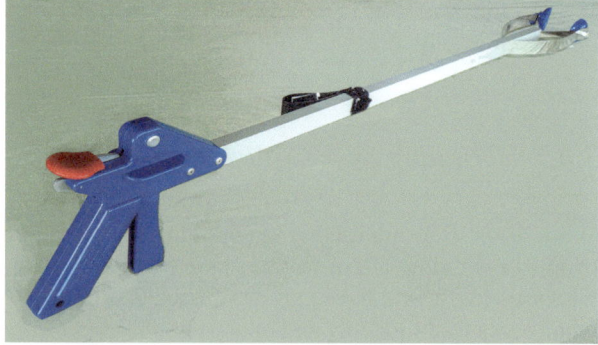

than the back of the path (or both sites). Obstacle height, width, and the number of obstacles impact risk. Perceiving the fall risk is important as the walker can avoid the obstacle. This is aided by placing the lighting source in front rather than behind the walking path [17].

3.4 Home

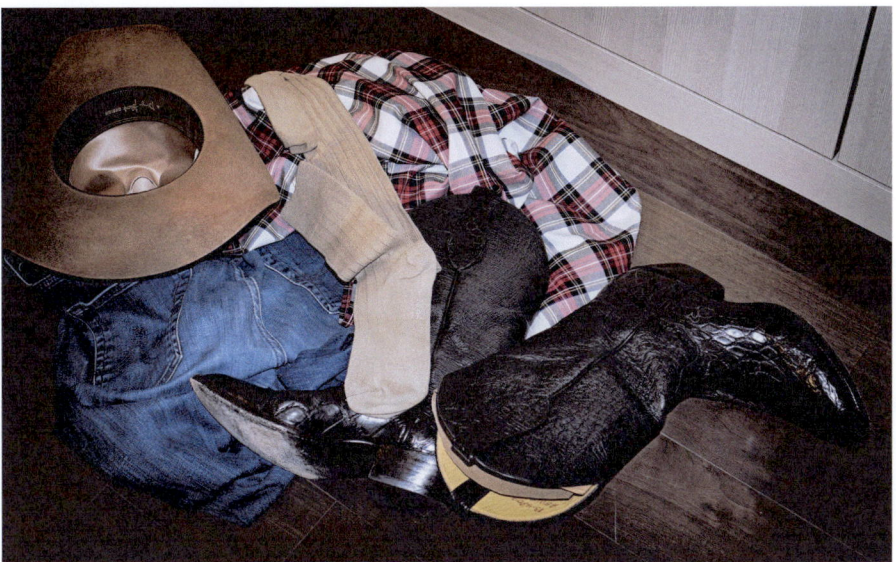

Fig. 3.10 While a cowboy probably will not get hurt tripping over cluttered clothing, an older individual may be at risk

3.4.8 Not Using the Night-Light

Night-lights are essential in preventing falls in limited balance because of age or chronic illness. As mentioned previously, balance is integrated between signals sent from the joints and muscles, the inner ear, and the eye. Around 20% of the nerve function in the eye integrates with the balance centers in the brain. Thus, what is safe during the day may become a threat at night. The likely scenario is that the individual with a full bladder awakens at night to use the bathroom and tries to walk to an adjacent room in darkness, having made the same trip hundreds of times. It is easy to lose balance and become disoriented enough to cancel one's familiarity with the path. A simple, strategically placed night-light can improve visibility so that the balance centers can receive signals from the eye (Figure 3.11).

3.4.9 Not Using a Walker, Cane, or Assistive Device

Assistive devices are often prescribed to elderly people with disability problems. These include impaired balance related to age, chronic conditions, or medications. Muscle weakness, neuropathy, and joint disorders can also impair balance and the ability to stand unattended. With poor vision, it is easy to trip over obstacles and lose footing. If the terrain is uneven or the floor surface is slick, the fall risk can be

Fig. 3.11 Night-lights are inexpensive and can reduce the risk of a fall

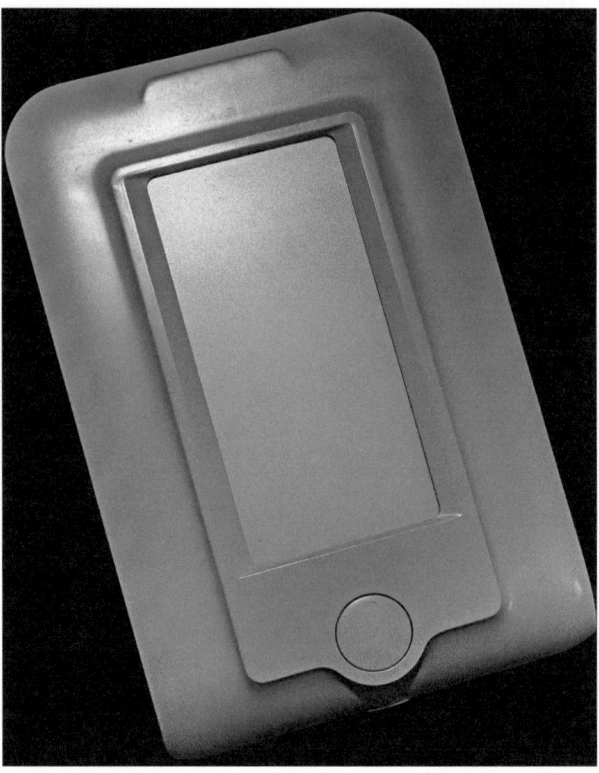

reduced using an assistive device such as a cane or walker. There are approximately 6.1 million in use (see Fig. 3.12).

Assistive devices can increase mobility and reduce the fear of falling. They aid with balance and redistribute weight. Standard canes can be used when only one upper extremity is needed for support but should not be used for weight bearing; an offset cane is helpful for weight support. A quadripod cane has four legs and increases stability.

Walkers are more appropriate if both upper extremities are needed for support. Walkers are especially useful in supporting persons with muscle weakness or poor balance. They can be devised with or without wheels. Those with wheels have the trade-off of allowing the gait pattern to flow better and not require lifting. They are less stable, however. Some walkers are made with four wheels. They are also known as rollators and are useful for those with adequate mental and physical function. While easy to propel, they are inappropriate for those with poor balance or cognitive impairment. They are fitted with brakes and may also be devised with seats and baskets. Proper fitting and training are necessary for the assistive device to provide adequate support. Many patients receive a device without either a recommendation or instructions from a medical professional. Improper device use can contribute to a fall if the person is destabilized in the process [18].

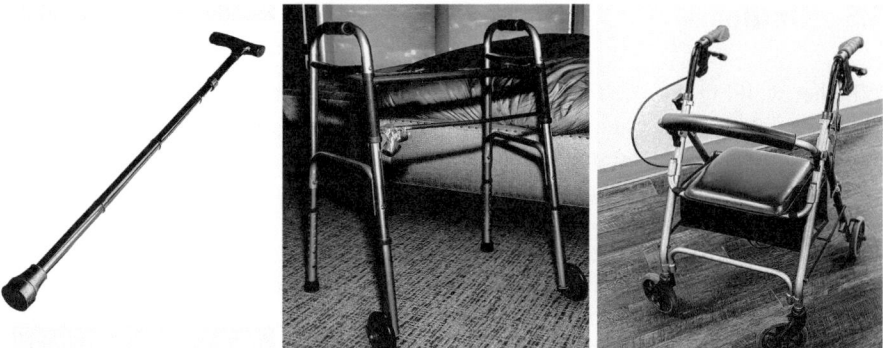

Fig. 3.12 The cane, walker, and rollator have specific uses. They must be maintained for safety. Accidents can happen if the caregiver and user are not properly trained

3.4.10 Wheelchair Safety

It is estimated that between 1.6 and 2.2 million Americans require a wheelchair. Since this population is already at high risk for a fall, it is not surprising that wheelchair injuries are common. Between 1991 and 2003, the number of wheelchair accidents that required emergency room visits doubled. 80.9% of these were tips and falls. 12.2% happened during transfers. In adults, 21.4% of injuries involved the head. Twenty-one percent were fractures. 81.5% of injuries occurred in an institution or hospital. 12.5% happened in the home. Many factors contribute to wheelchair-related falls. These include engineering flaws, the physical environment, and inappropriate training and use. Wheelchair maintenance also plays a role in accidents. Uneven terrain and home modifications may reduce the incidence of accidents [18].

3.4.11 Standing Too Quickly

Standing rapidly from a lying or sitting position can cause the blood pressure to fall if the autonomic nervous system is impaired. Also, volume depletion and blood pressure medications can result in a fall in blood pressure with any position change. This can also occur when changing position after exercising. This is known as orthostatic or postural hypotension and is a common cause of fall-associated fractures in the elderly. In addition, orthostatic hypotension can cause strokes, myocardial infarctions, and road accidents. Blood distribution in the body is influenced by gravity. When standing, less blood returns to the heart, and sensors tighten the blood vessel walls to stabilize the blood pressure. The blood pressure drops when these sensors or blood vessels do not work properly. This can result in light-headedness or passing out. Medications, diabetes, aging, immobility, and chronic blood vessel diseases can all cause hypotension when standing. Dehydration can make the problem worse [19].

3.5 Outdoors

Whether walking outside the house or hiking in a national park, certain principles guide a safe experience. Falls are one of the major hiking hazards. Finding medical assistance in national or state parks may be impossible as most do not have cell service. Satellite phones can be rented or purchased but require a line of sight that is not blocked by trees.

Fatigue and exhaustion can be treacherous if one overexerts oneself, especially if not staying hydrated. It is important to use hiking sticks and be aware of the terrain. Planning is important. Wear a hat, sunscreen, and appropriate clothing, and dress in layers. Use footwear with good traction to avoid slipping.

When walking in the dark, wear a headlamp. If walking in the neighborhood street, it will provide the light that can help you maintain your balance and avoid obstacles on the ground. Oncoming cars can also see and avoid you.

Hiking is far safer if elderly persons with compromised balance, an ankle or a knee disability to keep away from ledges and remain on designated hiking trails. Terrain can be quite rough when on a hike. When hiking over bridges, always note the guard rails (see Figs. 3.13, 3.14, and 3.15).

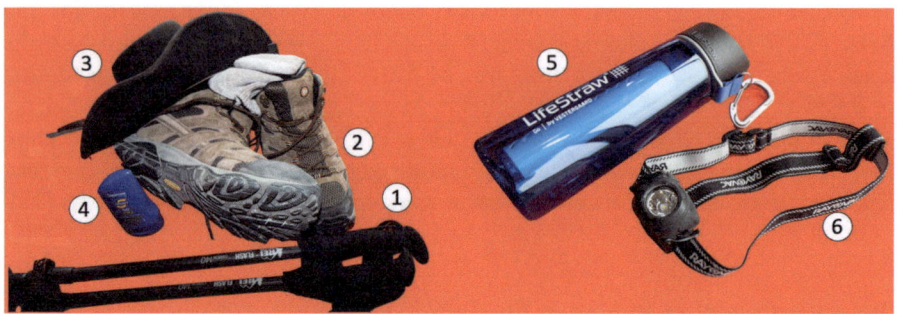

Fig. 3.13 Common errors when hiking. 1. Hiking without sticks. 2. Improper footwear. 3. Not wearing a hat. 4. Not using sunscreen. 5. Not taking and using a headlamp in darkness. 6. Carrying an inadequate water supply

3.5.1 Dangerous Rocks and Edges: No Support

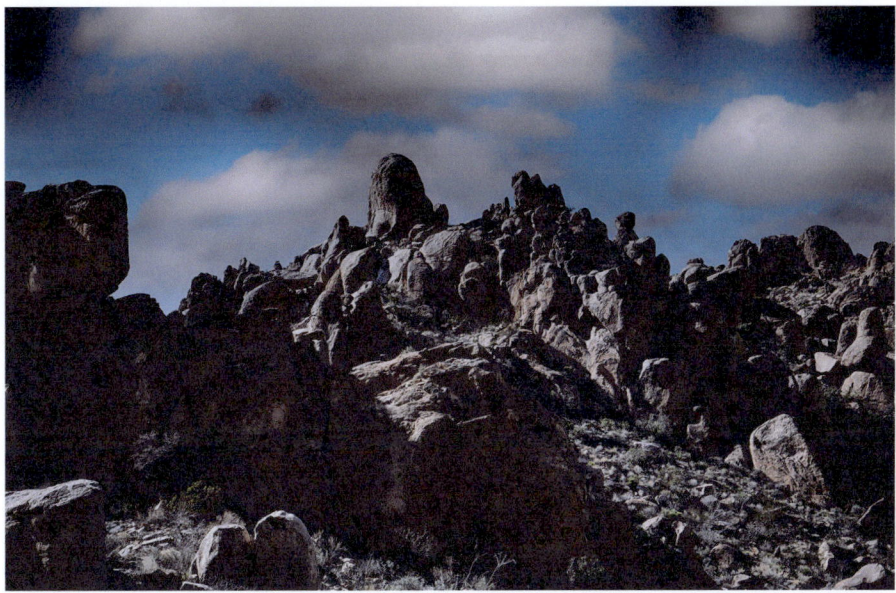

Fig. 3.14 Rocks and edges can be dangerous for those who have poor balance. Hikers need to plan according to their ability and skill

3.5.2 Lack of Guardrail Safety

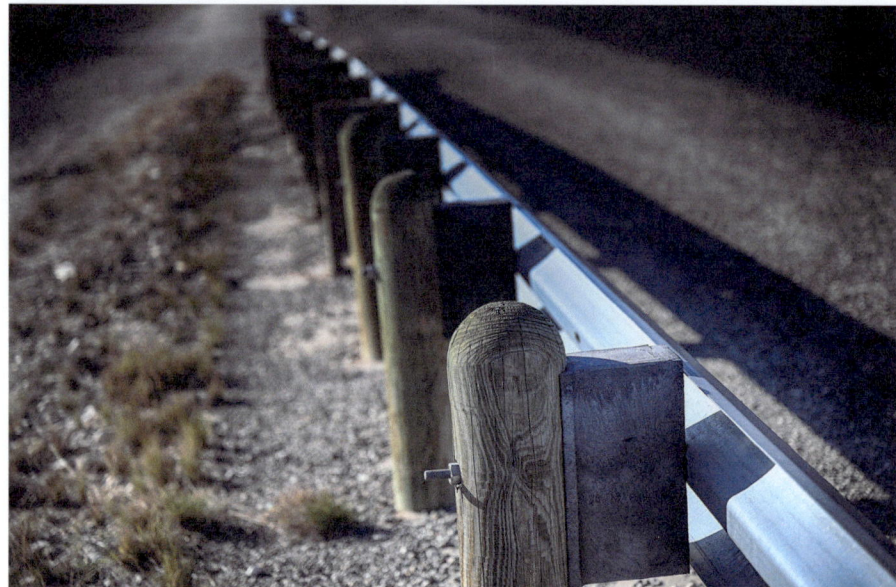

Fig. 3.15 Guardrails on bridges should not be crossed

3.6 Conclusion

Mechanical falls are often preventable by changes to the environment. This chapter has reviewed several reasons for mechanical falls. Eliminating these factors may reduce the risk of a fall in high-risk individuals. In a future chapter, we will review specific ways to reduce the fall risk in vulnerable populations.

References

1. Clemson L, Stark S, Pighills AC, Fairhall NJ, Lamb SE, Ali J, et al. Environmental interventions for preventing falls in older people living in the community. Cochrane Database Syst Rev. 2023;3(3):Cd013258. https://doi.org/10.1002/14651858.CD013258.pub2.
2. Kim D, Portillo M. Fall hazards within senior independent living: a case-control study. HERD. 2018;11(4):65–81. https://doi.org/10.1177/1937586717754185.
3. Ghahramani M, Stirling D, Naghdy F, Naghdy G, Potter J. Body postural sway analysis in older people with different fall histories. Med Biol Eng Comput. 2019;57(2):533–42. https://doi.org/10.1007/s11517-018-1901-5.

4. Blazewick DH, Chounthirath T, Hodges NL, Collins CL, Smith GA. Stair-related injuries treated in United States emergency departments. Am J Emerg Med. 2018;36(4):608–14. https://doi.org/10.1016/j.ajem.2017.09.034.
5. Mitchell SE, Aitken SA, Court-Brown CM. The epidemiology of fractures caused by falls down stairs. ISRN Epidemiology. 2013;2013:370340. https://doi.org/10.5402/2013/370340.
6. Lee HJ, Chou LS. Balance control during stair negotiation in older adults. J Biomech. 2007;40(11):2530–6. https://doi.org/10.1016/j.jbiomech.2006.11.001.
7. Sanchez-Ramirez DC, van der Leeden M, Knol DL, van der Esch M, Roorda LD, Verschueren S, et al. Association of postural control with muscle strength, proprioception, self-reported knee instability and activity limitations in patients with knee osteoarthritis. J Rehabil Med. 2013;45(2):192–7. https://doi.org/10.2340/16501977-1087.
8. Sudoł E, Małek M, Jackowski M, Czarnecki M, Strąk C. What makes a floor slippery? A brief experimental study of ceramic tiles slip resistance depending on their properties and surface conditions. Materials (Basel). 2021;14(22) https://doi.org/10.3390/ma14227064.
9. Oshima T, Ohtani M, Mimasaka S. Back hemorrhage in bath-related deaths: insights into the mechanism of bath-related deaths. Forensic Sci Int. 2020;308:110146. https://doi.org/10.1016/j.forsciint.2020.110146.
10. Katsuyama M, Higo E, Miyamoto M, Nakamae T, Onitsuka D, Fukumoto A, et al. Development of prevention strategies against bath-related deaths based on epidemiological surveys of inquest records in Kagoshima prefecture. Sci Rep. 2023;13(1):2277. https://doi.org/10.1038/s41598-023-29400-7.
11. Vladutiu CJ, Casteel C, Marshall SW, McGee KS, Runyan CW, Coyne-Beasley T. Disability and home hazards and safety practices in US households. Disabil Health J. 2012;5(1):49–54. https://doi.org/10.1016/j.dhjo.2011.10.003.
12. Levine IC, Lau ST, King EC, Novak AC. Consumer perspectives on grab bars: a Canadian national survey of grab bar acceptability in homes. Front Public Health. 2022;10:915100. https://doi.org/10.3389/fpubh.2022.915100.
13. Guitard P, Sveistrup H, Edwards N, Lockett D. Use of different bath grab bar configurations following a balance perturbation. Assist Technol. 2011;23(4):205–15.; quiz 16–7. https://doi.org/10.1080/10400435.2011.614674.
14. Amin K, Skyving M, Bonander C, Krafft M, Nilson F. Fall- and collision-related injuries among pedestrians in road traffic environment - a Swedish national register-based study. J Saf Res. 2022;81:153–65. https://doi.org/10.1016/j.jsr.2022.02.007.
15. Oxley J, O'Hern S, Burtt D, Rossiter B. Falling while walking: a hidden contributor to pedestrian injury. Accid Anal Prev. 2018;114:77–82. https://doi.org/10.1016/j.aap.2017.01.010.
16. Rosen T, Mack KA, Noonan RK. Slipping and tripping: fall injuries in adults associated with rugs and carpets. J Inj Violence Res. 2013;5(1):61–9. https://doi.org/10.5249/jivr.v5i1.177.
17. Li KW, Chen Y, Li N, Duan T, Zou F. Assessment of risk of tripping before and after crossing obstacles under dimmed lighting conditions. Work. 2020;66(3):551–9. https://doi.org/10.3233/wor-203197.
18. Bradley SM, Hernandez CR. Geriatric assistive devices. Am Fam Physician. 2011;84(4):405–11.
19. Dani M, Dirksen A, Taraborrelli P, Panagopolous D, Torocastro M, Sutton R, et al. Orthostatic hypotension in older people: considerations, diagnosis and management. Clin Med (Lond). 2021;21(3):e275–e82. https://doi.org/10.7861/clinmed.2020-1044.

Chapter 4
Consequences of Falls

4.1 Introduction

While a fall in the bathroom or bedroom might be minor for a younger and perhaps healthier individual, the same incident can result in serious injury for the elderly and vulnerable. Falls can lead to hospitalizations for fractures or head injuries. Rehabilitation can be difficult. In addition, falls can result in periods of immobility which worsen muscle and bone weakness. Loss of assuredness and the development of frailty can result from a fall. If the numbers of years of disability for all the falls that occurred in 2018 could be added together, it would amount to a staggering 38 million, based on statistics gathered on nonfatal falls by the World Health Organization (SOURCE: WHO).

Falls can lead to pain which can necessitate the use of pain medications. They can result in lacerations, muscle strains, and sprained or torn ligaments. This can amplify already existing balance problems. People who fall may lose independence, especially with a serious accident that requires a hospital stay. Hospitalizations can be associated with social isolation, immobility, a change in one's routine, and compromised quality of life. They can also culminate in burdening expenses. Falls also can have a psychosocial impact, especially if independence is compromised, and one must now have assistance in performing daily activities. They can lead to frustration and anxiety, depression, a loss of confidence, and lower levels of self-esteem.

A study in Canada showed that falls accounted for 85% of injury-related hospitalizations in persons over 65 years old and 77% of all injury-related hospitalizations. Although women fell more frequently than men, their survival rates after a fall were higher than those of men [1]. A study in Germany looking at falls occurring in nursing homes found that those with cognitive impairment had a 23.8% increase in the risk of sustaining a fall-related injury. The risk of injury was lowered by 16.7% when cognitively impaired individuals fell in a homelike environment rather than a traditionally organized facility [2]. Many people who fall are unable to get back up and consequently develop dehydration, muscle breakdown, and pressure sores.

4.2 Types of Falls

Examples of several types of falls are slipping on a slick surface, losing balance while carrying an object on the stairs, tripping over a loose object on the floor, or reaching for an object and stumbling. In a study that was done in Ireland, nearly half the falls were related to environmental factors, and most were from a height of less than 2 meters. As people age, their bones become more brittle and break easier. The limbs are injured in 42% of falls in the age group of 65 to 75, but this increases to 52% in the 85- to 95-year-old group. Spine injuries increase from 9% to 14% as people reach 95 [3]. Studies of falls show that 85.9% of injuries result from direct impact. The Irish study demonstrated that head injuries fell from 31% to 21% as people age. Video studies have demonstrated that impact is lowest to the head and highest to the hip and pelvic area [4].

Mortality and disability also rise in persons ≥65, with 10.9% dying and only 25% recovering following an injurious fall [3].

4.3 Head Injuries

Head injuries can refer to any scalp, brain, or skull fracture and range from mild to severe. In the elderly, they are most likely the result of a fall. Their impact ranges from a minor pain episode to severe disability. 64.2% of falls are mechanical. They are related to slipping on a slick surface, stumbling into an unexpected object on the floor, or colliding with another person. 16.6% of falls that require hospitalization happen when people lose their balance on the stairs, and 10.2% involve furniture. 4.1% of falls are related to ladders and scaffolds. Most hospital-related falls occur in the home. 13% of hospitalizations because of fall-related head injuries result in death [5].

4.3.1 Concussion

A brain concussion is characterized as a type of traumatic brain injury (TBI) that occurs when the brain is suddenly jolted inside the skull. There are 1.7 million patient visits to emergency rooms yearly for TBIs, mostly due to motor vehicle accidents [6]. TBIs can also occur after a fall. In the elderly, a fall is the most common reason for a TBI. Concussions occur in 24.1% of TBI admissions to the emergency room [5].

In a fall, hitting the head on a hard surface can cause a concussion. Some patients experience a headache, dizziness, nausea, disorientation and confusion, and a transient lapse in memory. The prognosis after a single concussion is generally good. There is concern that athletes who sustain several concussions during the course of their careers may develop chronic traumatic encephalopathy.

4.3.2 Brain Contusions

Sometimes the head impact is severe enough to cause a brain contusion. This can be severe and associated with brain hemorrhage. Brain contusions can progress and expand. Since blood is highly toxic to brain tissue, the area under the hemorrhagic contusion loses function. This is worsened in persons taking blood thinners. Brain contusions can cause permanent damage and result in disability or death.

Brain contusions are associated with motor vehicle accidents, falls, assaults, sports and recreation, cycling, blast injury, domestic violence, and child abuse. The injury is usually in the frontal and temporal lobes [7].

4.3.3 Skull Fractures

The blunt force of a sudden impact can cause a break in the skull bones surrounding and protecting the brain. Fractures may occur when the head hits the pavement, a hard floor, or furniture. The break can be mild and result in little residual damage. If severe, the break can be associated with bleeding and brain damage. It can lead to an infection and seizures. After a skull fracture, the skull may appear depressed or dented. In other cases, a lump may appear. The person may be disoriented and dizzy. Nausea, vomiting, and loss of consciousness with blood or clear fluid running from the ears or nose may occur with substantial injuries. A severe fall that injures the base of the skull may result in a fracture, bruises around the eyes, and clear fluid draining from the nose or ears. Sometimes the bleeding from a skull fracture takes hours to days to develop. Bleeding can also be chronic.

4.3.4 Hematomas (See Fig. 4.1)

Severe head injury can cause a blood collection to form. The blood collection is called a hematoma, and its location and severity depend on many factors, including brain anatomy. The brain is protected by a three-layer covering called the meninges. It is first encased in a heavy sheathlike material called the dura, which is directly under the skull. Below the dura is a middle layer called the arachnoid mater. The

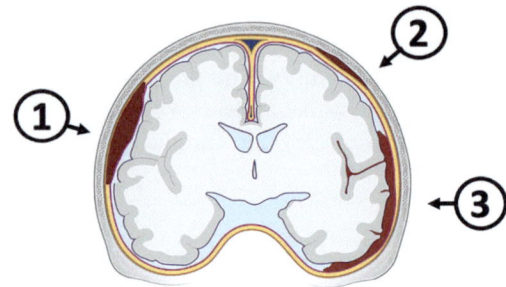

Fig. 4.1 Types of hematomas that can occur after a fall. Figure created with Adobe Photoshop and BioRender.com

1. Subdural hematoma
2. Epidural hematoma
3. Subarachnoid hemorrhage

arachnoid layer does not have nerves or blood vessels. Underneath the arachnoid layer is the inner layer, the pia mater. Cerebrospinal fluid circulates between these two layers. The pia contains many blood vessels and supplies the outer surface of the brain with oxygen and nutrients.

Extradural Hematoma

An extradural (also known as epidural) hematoma happens when blood collects outside of the dura, in the space between the bone and the outer part of the dura. Most are on the side of the head. This life-threatening emergency occurs when a meningeal artery bursts or a vein near the skull is lacerated by the injury. It is commonly associated with skull fractures. In 14 to 21% of injuries, there is an initial loss of consciousness and then a transient recovery followed by a complete loss of consciousness as the hematoma expands. A severe hematoma can compress the brain, forcing it to squeeze through the opening of the skull, compressing the brain stem and its vital blood supply. This can lead to permanent brain injury and death [8].

This type of injury is most likely related to motor vehicle accidents and assaults. It can also occur with falls. It is less common in the older population.

Subdural Hematoma

A subdural hematoma occurs when the veins from the brain are injured and drain in the space under the dura and on top of the arachnoid space.

Subdural hematomas make up 42.9% of hospitalizations with head injuries in persons over 85 years old [5].

Minor trauma can lead to a subdural hematoma even though there are no symptoms. This hematoma expands very slowly and initially presents as a headache. It can progress to confusion and paralysis. The diagnosis should be suspected in people who have any neurological changes after falling and hitting their head. The diagnosis can be made with a CT scan [9].

Subarachnoid Hematoma

A subarachnoid hemorrhage (SAH) occurs when blood collects between the pia mater and the brain. These can occur because of trauma but can also result from a ruptured aneurysm. They can also happen when an artery and vein do not develop properly, and flow is abnormal. This is called an arteriovenous malformation. A SAH commonly presents with a headache and a severe stiff neck, vomiting, and nausea. It is a medical emergency and account for 12.7% of all fall-related hospitalizations among the elderly.

4.4 Spinal Cord Injuries

The backbones are a major site for fractures in the elderly. While they compose only 5% of fractures in the 50- to 54-year-old age group, vertebral fractures comprise 50% of the fractures that are seen in persons between 80 and 84 years old [10]. Falls account for 28.9% of spinal cord injuries. This contrasts with assaults that are 2.9% and motor vehicle accidents that are 40.4%. They can lead to a neck injury that prolongs the hospitalization, increases the costs of healthcare, and can even be life-threatening. The rehabilitation of a person who sustains a spinal cord injury depends upon not just the extent of the injury but the disability, use of pain-relieving medications, and age [11].

4.5 Fractures

Fractures are common in the elderly because of osteoporosis, the loss of mineralization of the bone. Demineralized bone cannot support the body weight well and with impact easily breaks. There are nearly three million osteoporotic fractures each year. They cause pain, immobility, and loss of function and independence. Their recovery can be slow, and they often result in death. The typical long bone has two parts—the cortical or compact part and the spongy part known as the trabecular bone. The cortex is dense, and the spongy bone resembles a honeycomb (see Fig. 4.2 and 4.3). The bone has several different types of cells. One type, the osteoblast, makes bone. The osteocyte maintains it. A layer of bone lining cells helps control the sending of signals to either make or resorb cells. Osteoclasts break bones apart so that the minerals can be used for remodeling. Bone loss for men is around 0.3% per year and for women is 0.5% per year. In the postmenopausal years, it can increase to 5–6% yearly. The spongy trabecular or cancellous bone has a horizontal crosslink and a vertical beam structure. Both are important. When osteoporosis affects the horizontal parts of the bone, the beams become unsupported [12].

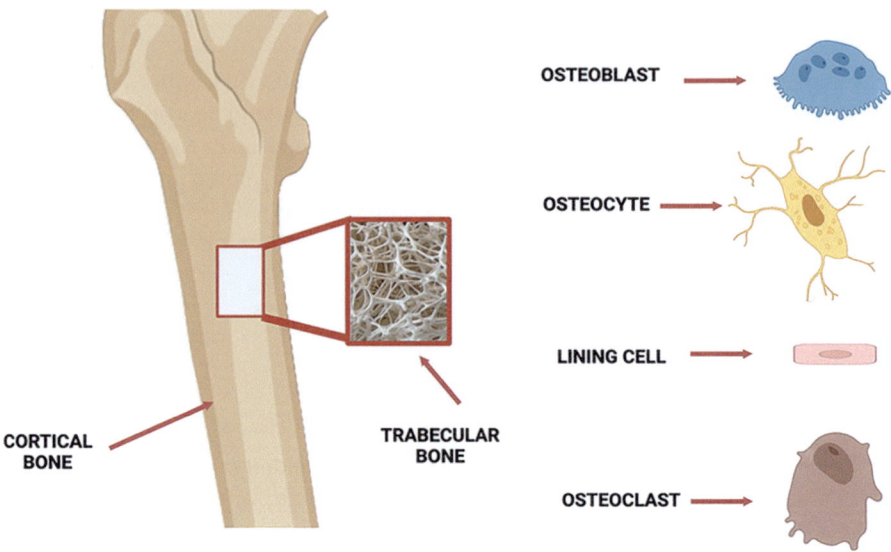

Fig. 4.2 Bone can be spongy with a honeycomb appearance. This is called cancellous or trabecular bone. Cortical bone is denser. Different cells have different jobs (see text). Created with Adobe Photoshop and BioRender.com

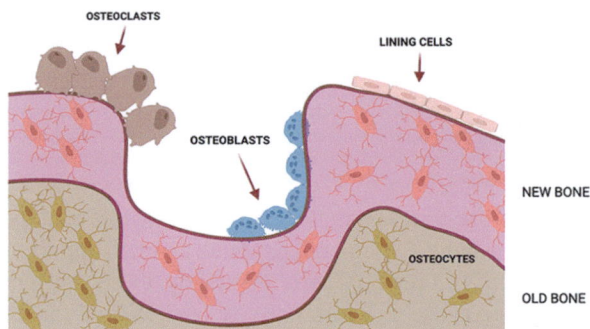

Fig. 4.3 Bone cells control the laying down and resorbing of bone. This is known as remodeling and is necessary for bone growth and maintenance. As persons age, the resorption increases proportionate to the laying down of bone. Created with Adobe Photoshop and BioRender.com

4.5.1 Vertebral Fractures (See Fig. 4.4)

Vertebral fractures are breaks in the bones in the back. They are among the most common fractures in the elderly. They also predict the risk of a subsequent hip fracture. Falls account for 30 to 50% of hip fractures. In a study made in persons who were ≥ 65 years old, lived at home, and sustained a new vertebral fracture after a fall, just over 50% of fractures occurred in the lower back (53.8% male and 52.8% female), while 29.5% of males and 35.6% of females had breaks in the thoracic spine—the part connected to the ribs. Men more commonly had neck fractures,

4.4 Fractures

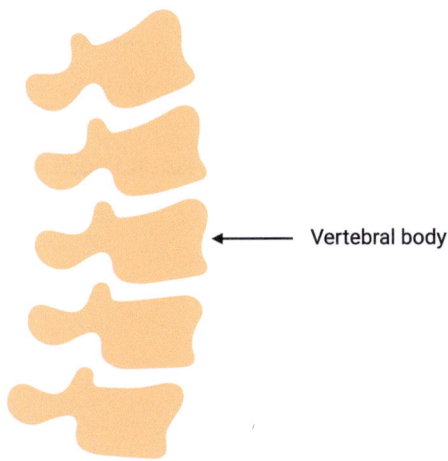

Fig. 4.4 The lower back—backbones. There are three sets of back bones—the neck or cervical bones, the chest or thoracic bones, and the lower back or lumbar vertebrae. Created with BioRender.com

14.1% compared to 7.8% of women. The tailbone was involved in 2.4% of men and 3.8% of women.

Vertebral fractures occur more often during indoor activities. Features associated with falls that resulted in vertebral fractures included toileting, slipping, stepping down, and falling backward or sideways. Women are more likely to fall when stepping down, getting out of a chair, and while walking. Men are more likely to slip, trip, and fall forward and fall on an uneven floor.

Falls on stairs or secondary to tripping occur less than 10% of the time [10].

4.5.2 Hip Fractures (See Fig. 4.5)

The hip or pelvis is connected to the thigh bone or femur with a ball and socket joint. The ball part of this joint is connected to the femoral shaft by a more narrow region of the bone called the neck. It is the neck that breaks with injury and which is referred to as a hip fracture. At least 95% of hip fractures in the elderly result from a fall, even though falls cause hip fractures only 1 to 2% of the time. Falls that produce hip fractures occur from a standing position with direct impact on the hip leading to a fracture at that point. The risk of a hip fracture is highest if falling sideways. The hip is among the first three parts of the body to hit the ground. It is the first bone to hit the ground in 17% of cases, the second in 40%, and the third in 43% of cases. In 67% of cases, the upper limb, either the hand or elbow, precedes the hip in hitting the ground. In 60% of hip fractures, the knee hits the ground before the pelvic impact. An assistive device lowered the risk of a hip fracture [13].

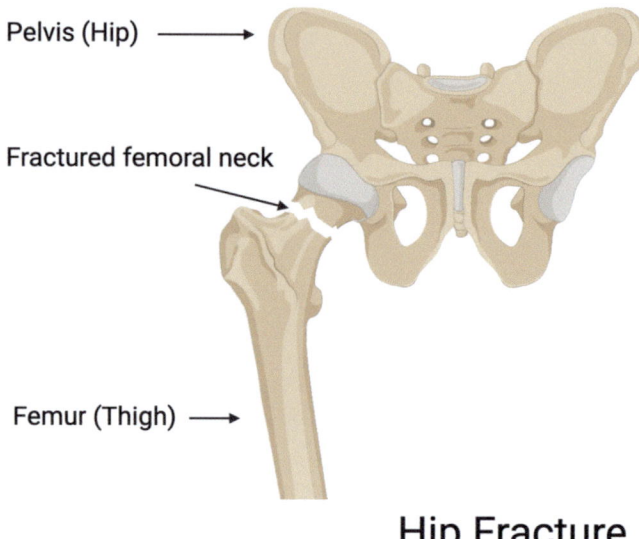

Fig. 4.5 A hip fracture most commonly results from a fall in an elderly person. Created with BioRender.com

4.5.3 Other Fractures

Forearm fractures generally occur around age 65, 10 years older than vertebral fractures. Hip fractures in women occur at the mean age of 82 years. In men, forearm fractures occur around age 54, 12 years younger than vertebral fractures. Hip fractures occur around the age of 78 [14]. Femoral shaft fractures can occur in the elderly with ground-level falls, particularly when osteoporosis is significant [15]. Although using skeletal traction may be a temporary measure to stabilize a femoral fracture, most femoral shaft fractures will require surgery [16, 17].

4.6 Conclusion

Falls often lead to injuries, many minor but some serious. The severity depends on the age and extent of underlying bone disease. Most falls in the elderly are from a height less than 2 meters and involve either a slip on a slick surface, tripping over an obstacle, falling while changing position, or walking. Falls can result in fractures to the back, neck, or hip. Head injuries many also occur and can lead to bleeding inside the skull.

References

1. Johnson S, Kelly S, Rasali D. Differences in fall injury hospitalization and related survival rates among older adults across age, sex, and areas of residence in Canada. Injury. Epidemiology. 2015;2(1):24. https://doi.org/10.1186/s40621-015-0056-1.
2. Zimmermann J, Swora M, Pfaff H, Zank S. Organizational factors of fall injuries among residents within German nursing homes: secondary analyses of cross-sectional data. Eur J Ageing. 2019;16(4):503–12. https://doi.org/10.1007/s10433-019-00511-3.
3. Lesko K, Deasy C. Low falls causing major injury: a retrospective study. Ir J Med Sci(1971). 2020;189(4):1435–43. https://doi.org/10.1007/s11845-020-02212-8.
4. Komisar V, Dojnov A, Yang Y, Shishov N, Chong H, Yu Y, et al. Injuries from falls by older adults in long-term care captured on video: prevalence of impacts and injuries to body parts. BMC Geriatr. 2022;22(1):343. https://doi.org/10.1186/s12877-022-03041-3.
5. Harvey LA, Close JC. Traumatic brain injury in older adults: characteristics, causes and consequences. Injury. 2012;43(11):1821–6. https://doi.org/10.1016/j.injury.2012.07.188.
6. Laker SR. Epidemiology of concussion and mild traumatic brain injury. PM R. 2011;3(10 Suppl 2):S354–8. https://doi.org/10.1016/j.pmrj.2011.07.017.
7. Kim SH, Kim S, Cho GC, Lee JH, Park EJ, Lee DH. Characteristics of fall-related head injury versus non-head injury in the older adults. BMC Geriatr. 2021;21(1):196. https://doi.org/10.1186/s12877-021-02139-4.
8. Khairat A, Waseem M. Epidural Hematoma. StatPearls. Treasure Island (FL): StatPearls Publishing. Copyright © 2023, StatPearls Publishing LLC.; 2023.
9. Traynelis VC. Chronic subdural hematoma in the elderly. Clin Geriatr Med. 1991;7(3):583–98.
10. Yu WY, Hwang HF, Chen CY, Lin MR. Situational risk factors for fall-related vertebral fractures in older men and women. Osteoporos Int. 2021;32(6):1061–70. https://doi.org/10.1007/s00198-020-05799-x.
11. Kennedy P, Cox A, Mariani A. Spinal cord injuries as a consequence of falls: are there differential rehabilitation outcomes? Spinal Cord. 2013;51(3):209–13. https://doi.org/10.1038/sc.2012.124.
12. Falaschi P, Marsh D, editors. Orthogeriatrics: the management of older patients with fragility fractures. Cham (CH): Springer. Copyright 2021, The Editor(s) (if applicable) and The Author(s). This book is an open access publication; 2021.
13. Yang Y, Komisar V, Shishov N, Lo B, Korall AM, Feldman F, et al. The effect of fall biomechanics on risk for hip fracture in older adults: a cohort study of video-captured falls in long-term care. J Bone Miner Res. 2020;35(10):1914–22. https://doi.org/10.1002/jbmr.4048.
14. Melton LJ 3rd, Amin S. Is there a specific fracture 'cascade'? Bonekey Rep. 2013;2:367. https://doi.org/10.1038/bonekey.2013.101.
15. Johnell O, Kanis J. Epidemiology of osteoporotic fractures. Osteoporos Int. 2005;16(Suppl 2):S3–7. https://doi.org/10.1007/s00198-004-1702-6.
16. Femoral LJ, Fractures S. In: Eltorai AEM, Eberson CP, Daniels AH, editors. Essential orthopedic review: questions and answers for senior medical students. Cham: Springer International Publishing; 2018. p. 145–6.
17. Martel DR, Tanel MR, Laing AC. Impact attenuation provided by older adult protective headwear products during simulated fall-related head impacts. J Rehabil Assist Technol Eng. 2021;8:20556683211050357. https://doi.org/10.1177/20556683211050357.

Chapter 5
Assessing Risk and Preventing Nonmechanical Falls

5.1 Introduction

In the first part of this book, we went through a deep dive into falls, helping us appreciate the medical and environmental circumstances associated with falling, as well as the consequential injuries that can occur. Now, we will develop a process to avert or reduce the damage that falls cause. The book's ultimate mission is to reach beyond purely understanding risks and mechanisms and to support preventing falls and fall-related injuries from ever happening. This may be daunting, even impossible, but only through awareness, research, and the implementation of the best ideas and practices can we move forward along a continuum. This chapter will highlight the materials taken from studies and trials that have been proven successful in persons who have been identified as having a high risk for a fall because of underlying medical disorders. The processes offered here may be tailored to one's individual needs. Strategies work best when they include efforts to reduce hazards and create a safe environment and will be further discussed in the following chapter.

When it comes to prevention, we work best as a team. This includes those of us involved directly in health care, such as physicians, nurses, physician assistants, nurse practitioners, social workers, dietitians, and medical assistants. Partnering health professionals include physical therapists, personalized trainers, occupational therapists, pharmacists, and balance-center professionals. We rely on patients and their families, along with caregivers, to incorporate fall prevention into their culture. Several agencies and health organizations are involved in the fall prevention process and have developed recommendations, tools, and resources. We will start with one of the most valued health resources, STEADI.

5.2 Assessment

The Centers for Disease Control and Prevention (CDC) has developed a useful three-step resource to screen, assess, and intervene to reduce adult fall incidence. Known as STEADI, the program is readily accessible from the CDC website.

Step 1 Screen for Fall Risk
The CDC asks and scores individuals using the following 12 questions:

1. I have fallen in the past year.
2. I use or have been advised to use a cane or walker to get around safely.
3. Sometimes I feel unsteady when I am walking.
4. I steady myself by holding onto the furniture when walking at home.
5. I am worried about falling.
6. I need to push with my hands to stand up from a chair.
7. I have some trouble stepping up onto a curb.
8. I often have to rush to the toilet.
9. I have lost some feeling in my feet.
10. I take medicine that sometimes makes me feel light-headed or more tired than usual.
11. I take medicine to help me sleep or improve my mood.
12. I often feel sad or depressed.

https://proptbalance.com/wp-content/uploads/2018/09/document9.pdf- One can download and take the simple test. One is not considered a fall risk if the score is <4, and there has not been a recent fall.

Step 2 Assess the Individual for Modifiable Risks and Fall History
In general, falls are likely to occur again if there has been a history of recent falls. Patients who are unsteady when standing and when walking have a legitimate fear of falling and should be considered to be high risk.

If a person's score is ≥4 or they have a recent history of a fall, there are eight steps that can be taken to identify modifiable risk factors. These are covered in this and the next chapter:

- Assess gait strength and balance (see Table 5.1 and Fig. 5.1).
- Timed Up & Go.
- 30-second chair stand
- 4-stage balance test.
- Medications that increase fall risk. One criterion to consider is Beers Criteria.
- Ask about potential environmental hazards.
- Measure the blood pressure lying and standing to determine if postural hypotension is present.
- Check vision for acuity.
- Assess feet and footwear.
- Assess vitamin D intake.
- Identify other diseases and conditions that could cause falls or make them worse (comorbidities).

5.2 Assessment

Table 5.1 Assessment of gait strength and balance – (CDC STEADI)

Time up & go (TUB)		
Assesses mobility		
Equipment: Stopwatch app on smart phone and chair		
1. Stand up from a chair.		
2. Walk to a line 10 feet away at a normal pace.		
3. Turn around and walk back.		
4. Sit back down.		
5. Record time.		
Patients should wear regular footwear and can use their walking aid if necessary. The attendant stays with the patient for safety. If TUG takes ≥ 12 seconds, it indicates a fall risk.		
https://www.cdc.gov/steadi/pdf/TUG_test-print.pdf		
30-Second Chair Stand		
Tests leg strength and endurance.		
Equipment: Stopwatch app on c and chair		
1. Stand up from a chair with arms folded across the chest		
2. Then sit back down		
3. Repeat for 30 seconds		
4. Record time		
Below average scores indicate a fall risk.		
Age	Men	Women
60–64	<14	<12
65–69	<12	<11
70–74	<12	<10
75–79	<11	<10
80–84	<10	<9
85–89	<8	<8
90–94	<7	<4
https://www.cdc.gov/steadi/pdf/STEADI-Assessment-30Sec-508.pdf		

Step 3 Intervention Tailored to Identified Risk Factors

If the screening determines that an individual is not a fall risk, one should still be educated about falls and fall prevention and participate in an exercise or fall prevention program. Reassessments should be done annually. If a person in this category does fall, a reassessment can determine modifiable risk factors and necessary interventions.

If the risk score is ≥ 4 or there has been a recent fall, the CDC has built in a set of recommendations for each of the eight factors above. The flow of these chapters deviates from the original CDC outline, but these and other recommendations have been incorporated into the discussions in this and the next chapters.

1. Gait, strength, and balance abnormalities.
2. Risky medications.

4-stage balance test
Assesses static balance **Equipment: Stopwatch app on smart phone** • Stand next to and steady the patient . • Time the patient standing in each of the four positions below . • Move to the next position if the patient holds a position for 10 seconds without moving   their feet or requiring support. • If not, stop the test.
1. Stand with feet side to side.
2. Place the instep of one foot so it touches the big toe of the other.
3. Tandem stand: Place one foot in front of the other – heel touching toe.
4. One leg stand .
An adult who cannot hold the tandem stand for 10 seconds or longer is at risk for a fall. https://www.cdc.gov/steadi/pdf/STEADI -Assessment-4Stage-508.pdf

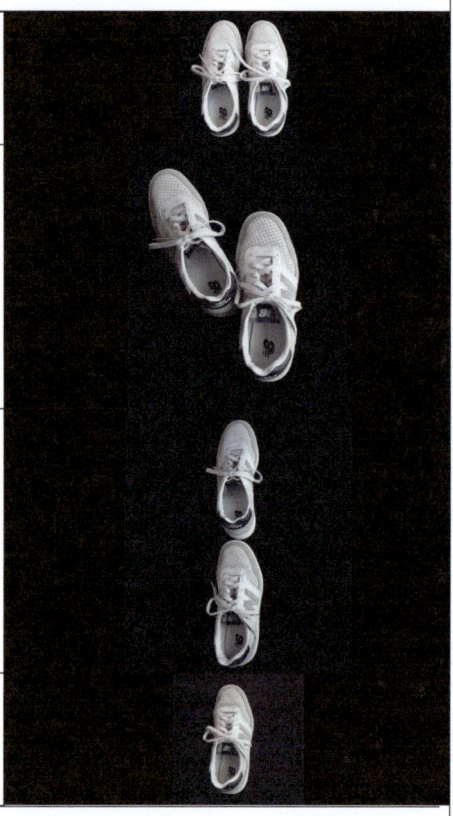

Fig. 5.1 Assessing balance - Shoe positions for 4-stage balance test

3. Environmental fall hazards.
4. Postural hypotension.
5. Abnormal vision.
6. Feet abnormalities.
7. Vitamin D deficiency.
8. Comorbidities.

5.3 Preventing Falls in Category 1: Frailty, Cognitive Decline, and Neurologic Deficit

Randomized trials to assess the impact of the intervention on falls in the elderly demonstrated that muscle strengthening and balance training were effective. Tai chi group exercise intervention also lowered the risk of falls. A fall is generally a "perfect storm" – with many of the risk factors at play working together to culminate in a weak and deconditioned person, perhaps with inner ear difficulties, either slipping or stumbling, then losing footing, and falling. The part of the body, the impact force, the surface characteristics, and the condition of the bones determine the nature and seriousness of the injury. Thus, targeting as many risks as possible decreases the chance of an injury.

Patients with disorders in this category generally will require assistance with the activities of daily living, including mobilization. They will be followed by a team of doctors and other health professionals, often including a licensed physical therapist. Assistive device prescriptions will likely be necessary, and it is important that the patient and caregiver understand its proper use. When vision, strength, balance, and gait are compromised, it is also important to ensure that the environment is free of hazards that could cause a slip or a stumble. Chapter 6 will highlight these preventive measures.

5.3.1 Frailty

The chance for a perfect storm is escalated with frailty, as well as with cognitive decline, a neurologic deficit, or aging. Many patients in this broad category are limited in their ability to perform the activities of daily living. They may also eat poorly and get little physical activity. Some have underlying medical conditions like arthritis, visual disturbances, diabetes, kidney disease, or heart failure. Depression, chronic pain, and sleep disorders contribute to falls and present risk reduction opportunities. Since many factors cannot be reversed, the objective is to focus on those that can.

Frailty is complex because it is not just dependent on age but factors such as the presence of dementia, blood vessel disease, and chronic disorders. After an assessment and a diagnosis of frailty, an action plan can be set up with the doctor and other health-care providers, the family, and the patient. For some people, frailty is an exit strategy, and we must respect that it is often an end-of-life process. When addressing the frail patient, we must consider the underlying disorder, the diet, medications, and exercise routine. Proper nutrition support and vitamin D help repair bones. Whether balance and muscle strength can be improved depends upon the individual, but the studies suggest optimism. In reviewing some of the randomized research studies in the medical literature, when compared with doing nothing, exercise and fall intervention programs reduce fall incidence [1, 2]. In one study, 305 elderly persons underwent aerobic exercise, strength training, balance, flexibility exercises, and a cool-down period for 1 year. At the end of the study, the frailty index score improved to a statistically significant degree [3]. Increased mobility and treating metabolic acidosis help strengthen muscles and reduce falling rates. Inexpensive safety hats and hip protectors may reduce impact injuries.

Although there are many options, the Otago Exercise Program has been especially effective in patients who are frail and has been validated; the entire exercise program will be published in Chap. **7**.

Otago Exercise Program (OEP)

This is a home-based fall prevention program that incorporates balance and strength exercises to prevent falls. It is designed to be administered by a licensed physical therapist and can be tailored to individual patients. It was initially designed for people over 80 years old with a history of falls and works best for frail adults. It is also useful for deconditioned adults and persons with chronic diseases. The CDC and National Center for Injury Prevention and Control (NCIPC) have adopted the program that was initially developed in New Zealand.

The program consists of five strengthening and 12 balance exercises, starting at 10 repetitions. They are to be performed three times a week. As one progresses, the number of repetitions can be increased, and ankle weights can be used. Walking for around1 h a week in two 30-min sessions or smaller and more frequent 10-min sessions is part of the program.

The program has been validated in four trials. It reduced falls by 30% to 66% and reduced fall-related injuries by 28%. About 70% of participants continued the program after the year study period ended [4].

5.3.2 Stroke

The best therapy for preventing stroke-related falls is to treat underlying stroke risks and emphasize prevention through blood pressure control and anticoagulation for atrial fibrillation. Two major causes of strokes are hypertension and atrial fibrillation. The Systolic Blood Pressure Intervention Trial (SPRINT) was a large clinical trial sponsored by the National Institute of Health (NIH). It enrolled 9,361 people who were diagnosed with hypertension. The aim of this 4-year study was to determine if strict blood pressure control (<120 mm Hg) would reduce the incidence of death, heart disease, and stroke. A total of 3,250 persons were ≥ 75 years of age. The study was stopped prematurely because it quickly revealed a 25% reduction in heart disease and strokes and a 27% decrease in death [5, 6]. This study demonstrated that regardless of age, the best way to prevent stroke was to control blood pressure.

In atrial fibrillation, the top chambers of the heart beat erratically. Normally, the heart is controlled by a conduction system that sends signals from one node to another and then through the entire heart. A node is like a station. When signals originate somewhere else in the heart's chambers, the heart beats erratically. Signals from the top part of the heart (atrium) cause atrial fibrillation, causing the heart muscle to pump blood irregularly. This can cause a decrease in the normal flow of blood, and a clot can form inside the heart. The heart can then pump the clot directly into the brain and cause a stroke. This is very damaging; atrial fibrillation is associated with a fivefold risk of stroke. Atrial fibrillation can be controlled with medications, but a very important part of therapy is the use of blood thinners. The newer blood thinners are far safer than what was available 10 years ago, and even safer blood thinners are in the pharmaceutical pipeline. These blood thinners can prevent a stroke. Although atrial fibrillation can be controlled by ablating areas in the heart that incite it, anticoagulation is still recommended for most patients who have had this procedure. A minimally invasive surgical procedure closes off the area of the heart that is associated with thrombus formation, the left atrial appendage. The WATCHMAN device closes this appendage and has been validated in numerous clinical trials to lower the risk of stroke caused by atrial fibrillation [7].

Brain-related injuries, deterioration, or tumors can result in serious brain-function loss. This invariably alters gait, balance, and mobility. Efforts should be made to rehabilitate patients to bring them to the highest level of function. This often takes a medical team that includes neurologists, internists, and specialists in rehabilitation. Sometimes the end result is limited. Patients with persistent gait and balance disorders will require an assistive device, either a cane, walker, or rollator. Those who cannot be rehabilitated to walk may require other types of assistance, such as wheelchairs. They will require close observation. Supervisory and care needs are based on the individual's ability to perform daily living activities.

After a stroke, the patient may be weak and debilitated. Also, there may be either complete or partial paralysis (paresis). Therefore, increasing patient endurance and fitness will need to be tailored to one's individual needs. After leaving the rehabilitation department, the patient may be so weak that daily activities are impossible to perform and walking outdoors is next to impossible. This is only made worse because adaptive movements needed to compensate for the paralysis and weakness. Exercise training is not only necessary after a stroke but must be sufficiently intense to strengthen the muscles that must adapt and take over the jobs of those muscles that are impaired. This also requires an increase in aerobic capacity. Strengthening the muscles also helps strengthen the bones after a stroke. Balance also needs to be relearned, but it is possible to achieve improvement with training [8–10]. Clearance of obstacles may be difficult after a stroke. Fall prevention will also necessitate ensuring safe pathways clear of clutter.

Fitness and Mobility Exercise (FAME)

In 2005, the Fitness and Mobility Exercise (FAME) Program for stroke was developed. Selective muscle strengthening exercises have improved post-stroke muscle strength in some patients. This program uses weights and elastic bands. The program considers that stroke patients often fall onto the side that is the weakest and that because of immobility, bones are fragile. Also, patients who require assistance when standing will need a caregiver who has been trained in assisting stroke patients to assist with the exercises. The program is designed for physical therapists and occupational therapists. It is a 1-h group program repeated two to three times weekly for at least 4 months. Self-directed home exercises, especially walking, should accompany the program. Patients should be screened by their physician and, if necessary, have a stress test to determine any cardiac limitations. The program starts with a 10-min warm-up period followed by stretching exercises. It then focuses on strength, balance, agility, and aerobic fitness. Most strength training exercises are done standing to force weight-bearing. Balance and agility include tai-chi-like movements. Chapter 7 discusses illustrated examples of the FAME program. The exercises start with two sets, five repetitions each, and progress to two sets of 10 repetitions. Patience is a critical attribute as post-stroke patients are slower; movements like the sit-to-stand exercise take significantly longer to perform [11]. Also, balance exercises should be taught and practiced in the context of everyday activities that involve standing, sitting, and reaching and moving objects.

The maximum target heart rate (MTHR) varies by age and historically was 220 minus the age in years. The newer MTHR is calculated by subtracting the age times 0.7 from 207. Thus, a 75-year-old person would have a maximum heart rate of around 155. If the resting heart rate for this individual is 75, then the heart rate reserve (HRR), the difference between the MTHR and the resting heart rate, is 80. The program starts with 40%–50% of HRR and progresses to 70%–80% of HRR. Thus, our 75-year-old would start with a target of $75 + 32 = 107$ to $75 + 64 = 139$ beats per minute. Participants should be screened with a treadmill test by a cardiologist, and this regimen should first be discussed with the doctor. The FAME program has been validated to improve stroke balance and muscle function, cardiovascular fitness, and bone density [12].

Many of the exercises are the same as in the Otago Exercise Program. The program also emphasizes socialization.

5.3.3 Dementia

Case presentation: An 81-year-old lady without a history of falls has been on hemodialysis for 3 years. She was recently diagnosed with Alzheimer's disease, but this is early, and she still functions very well. When coming in from the car with her daughter, she tripped over the doorstep and landed flat on her nose. She did not lose consciousness, and her daughter took her to the urgent care center. Other than a fractured nose and some bruising around her eyes, she had no injury. X-rays and computerized tomography (CT scan) of her head were normal. The following day, she went to her dialysis treatment. The nurses immediately recognized that she had fallen and started her dialysis therapy without using heparin, an anticoagulant.

5.3 Preventing Falls in Category 1: Frailty, Cognitive Decline, and Neurologic Deficit

Preventive steps: The patient's family, the emergency room, and the dialysis nurses did everything correctly concerning her care. Immediately after her fall, she was assessed and had a head CT scan to ensure that she was not developing a bleeding episode. The dialysis personnel held her heparin to safeguard against a bleeding problem.

Plan – This illustrative case demonstrates 10 steps that can be implemented to prevent falls in a patient who has become cognitively impaired.

1. Observation.
   - A potential head injury may not show any signs initially, but as the blood expands outside the blood vessels in the brain, it slowly becomes symptomatic, and behavior and personality may change. The family will watch for any changes and alert the doctors. Also, since she has fallen, she is at risk of falling again.

2. Risky medications.
   - In patients who require hemodialysis therapy, the routine anticoagulant therapy is not given as usual when there is concern that the patient has fallen, hit their head, and might have a brain injury.
   - Medications that cause sedation should be reviewed regularly and used only as needed. Medications that control the blood pressure may be necessary, but the blood pressure should be monitored closely both when lying and standing up. If there is a 10 mmHg drop in the systolic or top number or a 10 mmHg drop in the diastolic or bottom number, these medications should be adjusted.

3. Gait, strength, and balance abnormalities.
   - The patient's family will be taught the Otago Exercise Program to introduce to her. It will be introduced slowly, first with progressive strength building to help her with her gait and then balance training. Since she has dementia, the family will accompany and assist her with these exercises, which should take 30 mins thrice a week. On alternate days, she is encouraged to ambulate with assistance and her rollator.

4. Environmental fall hazards.
   - These tips are discussed in the next chapter, but here is a sneak preview. Ensure that any rugs are secure and that there are no obstacles on the floor for her to trip on. When possible, assist patients with dementia or gait disorders over potential "stumble steps." Grab bars should be installed in the bathroom so she does not slip on the wet floor after bathing. Nonslip bath mats will also help. Night lights along the path are essential if she must use the restroom at night.

5. Abnormal vision.

    - She will be referred to an ophthalmologist to check her visual acuity, to ensure that she does not have macular degeneration, cataracts, or glaucoma.

6. Feet abnormalities.

    - Patients who develop dementia may have trouble walking. An assistive device such as a walker or a rollator will help increase her confidence, ensure she is mobile, and protect her from falling again.

7. Nutrition and vitamin supplements.

    - Many patients with dementia lose their appetite. Food supplements may be necessary. The diet should be liberal enough that the food is tasty. The dietitian will work directly with her to find the foods that she enjoys the most.

8. Comorbidities.

    - The patient is currently on dialysis and is followed closely by a kidney specialist. The goals will be to ensure that waste products are effectively removed from the blood and that her body fluids are kept within the narrow therapeutic window. If she becomes too dry, she will faint, but if she has fluid overload, her heart will not pump sufficiently to move blood around and she will suffer from a lack of oxygen.

9. Reduce impact injury.

    - Since she is a fall risk, hip pads and a hat may prevent falls when walking outdoors. (See Figs. 5.2 and 5.3).

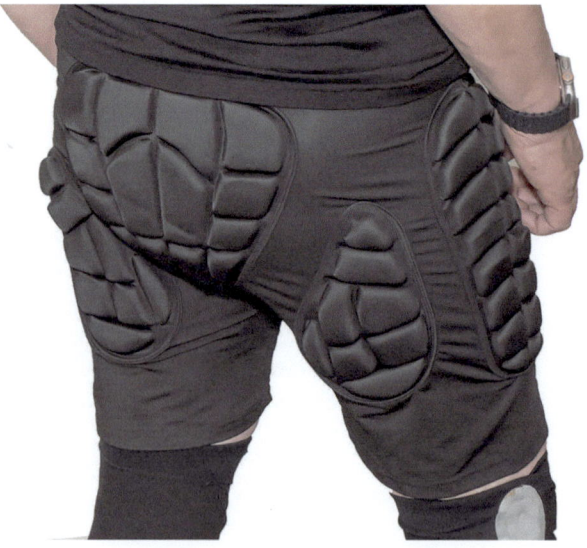

Fig. 5.2 Specially padded exercise shorts offer some protection from falls

5.4 Adjusting Medications to Prevent Falls

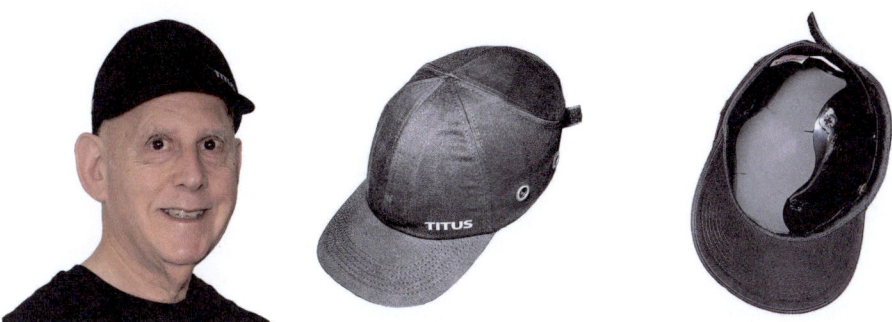

Fig. 5.3 What looks like an ordinary baseball hat has padding and a plastic inner lining to help protect the head in case of a fall

10. Other Tips.
    - Smartphones are now equipped with voice activation. Services like Siri or Alexa may be useful for her to reach out in case of danger and to alert loved ones and friends to keep track of her. Motion detectors can be worn and will identify when she has fallen. If she lives alone and falls in a bathroom, yelling for Siri to call help may save her life.
    - The family has been advised further to hold her liquids before bedtime so she will not have the urge to wake up at night to urinate.

5.4 Adjusting Medications to Prevent Falls

Fall-risk-inducing drugs (FRIDS) are important modifiable risk factors for reducing falls. In a combined review of several studies present in the medical literature, they increase the odds of a fall by 57%. Yet, untreated depression is also associated with a risk of falls, as well as with many other health issues in the elderly, including functional decline, decreased quality of life, and even suicide. Thus, the use of antidepressant therapy is common in the elderly; nearly 10% of persons are living in the community but are not residing in nursing homes. Nearly half of nursing home residents receive antidepressants. When antidepressants are deprescribed, the risk of sustaining a fall is lowered. The major category of antidepressants are selective serotonin reuptake inhibitors (SSRIs). They are associated with both nocturia and daytime drowsiness, both of which can increase the number of falls. SSRIs can also cause orthostatic hypotension and bradycardia, bone loss, Parkinsonism, nausea, and loss of appetite. Withdrawal from antidepressants is highly challenging for the physician and may lead to anxiety and a relapse of depression. If the benefit versus risk of an SSRI has not been determined, withdrawal should be carefully done over a period of weeks to months. To help assist providers with making decisions regarding the appropriate use of antidepressants in the elderly, a comprehensive tool,

Screening Tool of Older Persons' Potentially Inappropriate Prescriptions (STOPPFall) has been developed. There was consensus to stop drugs such as Valium, antipsychotics, opioids, antidepressants, and certain diuretics (water pills) [13].

The main reason to stop using a drug for diabetes is that low blood sugar can cause falls. However, many of the newer antidiabetic medications, such as the SGLT2 inhibitors, generally do not cause blood sugar to fall.

Water pills such as furosemide can cause a fall in blood pressure and the blood volume to decrease. The body must have a certain amount of fluid circulating in the bloodstream, and medications that eliminate salt reentry in the kidney can lower blood pressure. While this is the desired effect most of the time, it can lead to overly medicating and diuresing a patient, leading to a fall in the blood pressure when the patient stands. This results in unsteadiness and sometimes a fall [14].

5.5 Reducing Falls in Chronic Illnesses and Disorders

5.5.1 Age-Related Falls

Screening for falls is recommended each year for persons over 65 years old. The American Geriatrics Society and the British Geriatric Society have endorsed this recommendation. The CDC's STEADI Initiative, which was introduced earlier in this chapter, is an excellent program designed to assess risks and prevent falls. **https://pubmed.ncbi.nlm.nih.gov/29710141/**

A systemic review of the medical literature suggests that the focus on preventing falls should be on comorbidities, vitamin D levels, polypharmacy, frailty, sarcopenia, and home environmental fall hazards. Measures such as fall hazard reduction are only valuable when combined with other strategies such as an exercise program.

Exercise is the cornerstone of therapy in treating many age-related diseases, particularly cardiovascular, metabolic, and musculoskeletal disorders. Yet, training must be safe, effective, and fun to be accepted.

5.5.2 Comorbidities

Comorbidities are conditions or diseases that can either potentiate falling or make a serious injury more likely. Discussions of comorbidities constitute a major portion of this book because of the impact they have on both the fall event and its outcome. Certain conditions stand out and are being presented with an emphasis placed on preventive interventions.

5.5.3 Chronic Kidney Disease

Although the incidence of falls in patients with kidney disease is determined by age, other factors are also in play. A large number of medications dialysis patients take contributes to a fall risk. Depression and its therapy are also risks. Frailty, sarcopenia, decreased bone mineralization, and poor nutrition compound other risks. A CKD patient who falls likely will fall again. When the serum albumin level is low it reflects not just poor nutrition, but inflammation. A low serum albumin is a marker of chronic progressive disease and is a bad prognostic sign.

The rate of falls in dialysis patients is nearly 30%, with 70% requiring hospitalization. Around 11% of those will be hospitalized with a fracture, although head injuries and hip injuries are less frequent. This is fortunate as dialysis patients require an anticoagulant during treatment [15]. When a fall occurs in kidney disease patients, it doubles the risk of hospitalizations and death. Around 57% of falls occur when patients are ambulating [16]. Thus, advanced kidney disease patients should undergo yearly assessments. Gait and balance disorders may respond to balance training and Otago exercises. Additionally, the patient should be offered a rollator or walker with wheels. Of the comorbidities that are associated with falls, dementia is the major factor that is not modifiable. Some types of community-acquired pneumonia are preventable with vaccines.

Diabetes is common in kidney disease and an established cause of falls [17]. By the time diabetes damages the kidneys, it likely has damaged the nerves in the legs, the retina in the eye, and the heart muscle. It also decreases the ability of the stomach to move food down to the intestines and impairs the sensation of making urine. When it is advanced, diabetes causes the legs and feet to become numb to both heat and objects. Thus, burns from showers and baths that are too hot and severe bruises can be seen. Patients with advanced diabetes should never draw their own water for bathing and just use an infrared thermometer to ensure the bath or shower water is not too hot. It should not be more than a few degrees higher than your body temperature. Also, diabetics should never cut their own toenails and fingernails, as they are prone to infections.

Dialysis patients have problems with the acid content of their blood (metabolic acidosis), anemia or a low red blood cell count, inflammation, and too much phosphorus in the blood. Atrial fibrillation is also common. Many dialysis patients are on anticoagulants. Each of these conditions is regularly addressed by the doctors and team managing the dialysis patient.

The major problem associated with dialysis is the need to remove the volume of fluids that are gained between treatments. It is difficult to control the fluid gains that occur because the salt content of the diet makes us thirsty. Restricting dietary salt is recommended but understandably difficult. Over time, the heart beats against elevated blood pressure and into narrowed vessels because of the chronic damage of both blood pressure and chronic calcification. Forcing blood through narrowed blood vessels strains the heart muscle, and when it becomes damaged from wear and tear, scar tissue forms. Since this scar tissue conducts electricity poorly, the signals from the top part of the heart may not be sent throughout the heart muscle. An erratic heartbeat can appear. This is known as ventricular fibrillation and is a very common cause of sudden death.

In addition to this problem, wear and tear damages the heart muscle and causes heart failure. Treatment in dialysis patients involves limiting salt intake and weight gain between dialysis treatments. There is a narrow window for adequate therapy in dialysis patients. Too much fluid removal damages the heart, and too little fluid removal can leave burdensome salt and fluid on board [18].

5.5.4 Hypertension

Hypertension or high blood pressure is a risk factor for stroke and heart disease. High blood pressure also damages the kidneys, eyes, and blood vessels. It is controllable with medications, and evidence has shown that the better it is controlled, the lower the rate of stroke, heart disease, and even death. Major studies have now shown that lowering the blood pressure to under 120 mm Hg and even lower is associated with less death and heart disease, even in the elderly [19–21]. However, the survival curve is worse for frail persons over 80 years old who are taking several blood pressure medications [22]. In persons over 80 years old, the higher blood pressure may help preserve cognitive function.

Syncope is higher when the blood pressure is intensively treated. Falling is more likely to happen during the 15 days of starting antihypertensive therapy [23]. The risk of hip fractures can be associated with initiating treatment in the elderly [24].

Patients who are robust and healthy will benefit from intense blood pressure control, but patients who are frail should be cautious; it increases the risk of falls and death [25].

5.5.5 Diabetes

A study looked at 295,282 subjects and classified them into diabetes and non-diabetes who either exercised or did not. Falls were more common in diabetics, but the risk was over 20% higher in the inactive group [26].

5.5.6 Congestive Heart Failure

When the heart fails to supply the body's needs for oxygen and nutrients, the consequences increase the risk of a fall with a serious injury. Heart failure patients are often short of breath and can become weak, short of breath, lightheaded, and dizzy. Heart failure can be associated with irregular heartbeats and postural hypotension.

The diuretics that help reduce the fluid buildup associated with heart failure may lead to dehydration.

Exercising as tolerating to improve balance, endurance, and strength can help reduce the risk of falls. Also, if having any symptoms from medications, patients are advised to contact their physicians. Basic fall prevention procedures can help reduce mechanical falls. Measures to improve balance range from properly fitted shoes with good arch support to nonslip soles, and balance control will help prevent a fall. Any fall, even if minor, should be reported to the physician or health team so that a reevaluation can be planned.

5.5.7 Postural Hypotension

With position change, from 500 to 700 cc of blood shifts from the upper body, and the body normally adapts to maintain blood pressure. Damage to the nervous system, as with diabetes, dehydration, and medications that affect vascular tone or the nerve response to a position change can lead to a positional change in the blood pressure. When the systolic or top number drops over 20 mmHg or the diastolic (bottom number) drop is greater than 10 mmHg, a patient is said to have postural hypotension. This is also known as orthostatic hypotension. Orthostatic hypotension can cause light-headedness, dizziness, or fainting. It is a cause of chronic fatigue. The risk of developing symptomatic postural hypotension increases with age and is a common cause of falls. Medications that raise blood pressure and help treat postural hypotension include fludrocortisone and midodrine [27].

5.5.8 Sleep Disorders

Sleep Apnea

Case: A 68-year-old man with sleep apnea and a chronic lung disease associated with not eliminating enough carbon dioxide accidentally fell getting out of bed. He could not get back up, lying on the floor for several hours. As a result, he developed a severe muscle-breakdown injury that caused acute kidney injury.

Obstructive sleep apnea, the official term for sleep apnea, is associated with a lack of oxygen. This impairs posture and gait, increasing the fall risk. Obesity is associated with sleep disorders. It can interfere with upper airway structures and causes sleep apnea. This man had a body mass index of 50. Obesity also increases the difficulty of moving air in and out of the lungs. Additionally, with obesity, more oxygen is required, and more of the by-product of respiration, carbon dioxide ($CO2$), is produced. Since less oxygen is inhaled, the body suffers from a relative lack of oxygen. When $CO2$ is not exhaled properly, it causes a buildup of acids [28]. The respiratory drive is also affected by the balance of acids and bases in the body. It can also be affected if medications like diuretics cause a buildup of alkalis.

When he came to the attention of doctors, his kidney disorder was promptly treated, and he recovered. His sleeping and lung disorders were evaluated, and he was treated with a continuous positive airway pressure (CPAP) machine. He was then started on a physical therapy and exercise program that would help him both build muscle and correct his body mass index.

Nocturia

Nocturia is not a sleep disorder but a problem that affects around ten million people and is common in up to 1 out of 3 persons over the age of 30. By the age of 65, it affects over half the population. Around 48% of men and 30% of women have two episodes of nocturia each night [29]. Aside from the loss of sleep, nocturia is a fall risk. It accounts for a substantial number of falls and fractures, increasing the risk by 32% [30]. Yet, nocturia can be treated.

Some older men and women have an urge to rush to the bathroom. This can be a sign of an overactive bladder. When rushing to the toilet, especially at night, there is the risk of a fall. Men may have an enlarged prostate that also can cause nocturia.

5.5.9 Arthritis

We take for granted our bones and joints. As we age, we often develop degenerative arthritis. Proprioception is the natural ability that we have to know where we are, and it is worse with osteoarthritis. A loss of proprioception worsens arthritis, and arthritis impairs proprioception. Proprioception signals from the joints work along with vision and the inner ear to help us keep our balance and sense of position. When proprioception is poor, the gait is impaired, and unsteadiness leads not just to a fear of falling but to actual fall risks. Pain and muscle weakness accompany knee osteoarthritis, but with physical therapy to strengthen the quadriceps, pain, muscle strength, and proprioception can improve [31]. Patients with knee pain should consult their orthopedists and, when appropriate, get into a physical therapy program. When the program ends, a personalized trainer can take over to help you maintain quadriceps strength, control the pain through fitness, and improve proprioception.

5.5.10 Vision Disorders

Four major conditions can interfere with vision. Diabetic retinopathy is a major cause of blindness and can be treated when detected early. Physicians and clinics routinely examine patients to determine if the initial signs of diabetic retinopathy are present. Age-related macular degeneration (AMD) is hard to manage, but progress has been made, especially in reducing the risk of early AMD progression. The

area where the optic nerve begins is progressively damaged, leaving a large blind spot. Glaucoma can be easily detected through a simple eye exam – testing for intraocular pressures. Initially, patients will be asked to use eye drops each night. Other forms of therapy for glaucoma are also available and have been proven successful. Cataracts can worsen vision but can be removed by ophthalmologists. The procedure has been simplified with the use of robots. Making sure vision is optimal with regular checkups with the ophthalmologist can help reduce fall risks. Eyeglasses should be clean (not with tissue paper, it will scratch the glass) and worn when necessary.

Some medications, such as those in the family known as anticholinergics, can affect vision. Also, poor diabetes control can impact visual acuity.

5.5.11 Gait Retraining

Those who are debilitated or who have sustained an acute illness likely have difficulty walking properly. The ability to relearn proper gait technique depends upon the underlying disorder. As part of the follow-up convalescent visit, one should visit with the doctor to ensure clearance for exercise and get a referral to a physical therapist. The essential gait training exercises can be tailored to the patient's needs and are generally simple. The reader will be familiar with many of them. The Otago exercises described above help with gait training. Wearable sensors that measure body motion can provide the feedback needed to support training. This is true in both frail and healthy older adults [32].

A slow pace, loss of balance, short stride, little or no arm swing, scissor walking, wide-based gain, needing to steady one's self on the wall, shuffling gait, not using the cane or walker properly, and uncoordinated turning may indicate a neurological condition. Appropriate referral to a specialist may be needed.

5.5.12 Muscle Weakness

Muscle weakness is associated with falling. However, exercise training has been shown to improve the muscles. A study combining European researchers studied untrained healthy men who underwent high-intensity small-sided football training (soccer training) for 1 year. Blood samples and muscle biopsies were done and showed that markers for healthy glucose metabolism increased. These markers, adiponectin, AMPK, and mitochondrial messengers like SIRT1, all improved [33]. Although not for everyone, recreational soccer is now being recommended at a legitimate activity to improve the health and fitness of the elderly. The "Football in Medicine" platform offers scientific evidence and the large-scale implementation of evidence-based concepts from 35 peer-reviewed medical journals and over 150 scientific articles [34]. Patients are advised to consult their physicians before changing to heightened activity programs.

Sarcopenia is associated with type 2 diabetes and a high body fat percentage. Bioinformatic studies show the risk of sarcopenia is associated with alcohol intake, smoking, watching television, a high-salt diet, white bread, processed meats, neuroticism, falls, and fatigue. Muscles are protected by a high bone mineral density, serum testosterone levels, vitamin D levels, cognitive performance, education, physical activity, coffee drinking, and healthy diets (whole grains, potassium, magnesium, cheese, oily fish, protein, water, fruit, and vegetable intake). Resistance exercise induces the expression of genes that prevent sarcopenia [35].

5.5.13 Balance

Vertigo is a condition where there is a sensation of spinning caused by changes in the inner ear.

Persons who develop either hearing loss, ringing in the ears, or vertigo should see their physician. They may need an evaluation for hearing and inner ear disorders. If a balance assessment reveals abnormalities, a referral to a balance center is an excellent starting point to help regain function.

To recap from the previous chapter, the inner ear also controls balance. It contains three semicircular canals, fluid-filled curved tubes that are lined with sensitive nerve cells. As the fluid moves across the cells, signals are sent to the brain, which working like a giant computer, coordinates these signals along with those from vision and the joints. Together, these signals help us move or stand without feeling unsteady. Although a loss in the ability to hold one's balance is common with aging, it can be improved with training.

The Otago Exercise Program has been validated as improving the balance. In persons who are more robust, advanced exercises also fine-tune and improve balance (see Chap. 7). Tai chi (see Chap. 8) can also improve balance.

5.5.14 Peripheral neuropathy and Foot Disorders

Falls frequently occur in patients with neurological disorders. One such disorder, peripheral neuropathy, can occur in advanced diabetes and with cancer chemotherapy. It can damage the nerves that carry sensation to and from the arms and legs. This results in numbness, muscle weakness, and loss of coordination and balance. Neuropathy can be painful, and the medications used to control this pain can alter mental status. Exercise, strength training, and balance exercises that incorporate exercises into daily activities may help offset the negative influence of neuropathy. The impact of intervention varies with age, degree of debility, the degree of exercise, medications, and the presence of arthritis [36].

Special footwear, orthotic insoles, and arch supports may be necessary for some patients. A review of the medical literature demonstrated that podiatry interventions significantly reduce the incidence of falls in the elderly [37]. Podiatry interventions include ensuring patients have appropriate footwear, foot and ankle exercises, and podiatry care [38]. They may prescribe orthotics, specifically customized devices made from a foot impression. They support, align, and correct ankle and foot abnormalities. The benefits of orthotics can indirectly reduce falls by helping to increase comfort during walking and exercise.

5.5.15 Bone Loss

Osteoporosis is characterized by weak and fragile bones that fracture easily. It is common in the elderly and is associated with a fivefold increase in the risk of backbone fractures and 2–3 times the fracture of other bones. Medications that help treat osteoporosis are available, but the bones once again deteriorate once these drugs have been stopped. Universal recommendations include patient counseling, calcium, vitamin D supplements, monitoring, and coordinating post-fracture care with liaisons that can treat and rehabilitate patients. These guidelines recommend that once diagnosed, osteoporosis patients avoid cigarettes or excessive alcohol and that they be assessed for falls. Patients should start balance training, muscle-strengthening exercises, and safe movement programs, Fall risks such as sedating medications, polypharmacy, hypotension, and gait and vision disorders should be addressed and corrected. The home should be evaluated, and at-home fall hazards should be removed [39].

Although guidelines continue to recommend oral vitamin D supplements, there is evidence to support that vigorously exercising 3 h a week will raise vitamin D levels in men. Vitamin D supplementation may not be helpful alone, especially if the vitamin D levels are already sufficient. In addition to raising vitamin D levels, exercise is also associated with a 22% lower rate of heart attacks (myocardial infarction) [40].

Exercise is an important means of managing osteoporosis. Exercise can improve muscle strength and balance, ankle flexibility, muscle strength in the limbs and core, and the ability to get back up from the ground.

5.5.16 Volume-Related Disorders

A large 4-year study of 30,634 patients identified a positive association of dehydration with falls. Falls or death were positively associated with dehydration, loop diuretics, and with antipsychotic medications [41].

It is important to recognize the role that volume intake plays in maintaining health status. Diabetic patients are at high risk for dehydration because high blood sugar levels act as a diuretic. Many diabetic patients have abnormal kidneys that cannot retain fluids, and the neuropathy associated with diabetes destroys the body's ability to use the nerves to autoregulate the blood pressure. Neurological regulation of the blood pressure is normally done by a part of the nervous system called the autonomic nervous system, but this is damaged in diabetes. Maintaining adequate volume status is vital to protect diabetic patients from blood pressure drops.

Volume control through maintaining adequate hydration is a modifiable risk factor for falls in the elderly. If the body's fluid volume is decreased, it cannot rid the body of heat or support the blood pressure. Muscles are inefficient engines and generate around 70% of heat and only 30% of work. If that heat is not dissipated, then body tissues cannot function. The body relies on fluid intake to have ample resources of fluids for sweat. During times of heat stress, the kidneys try to concentrate the urine. However, elderly patients may have impaired kidney function and cannot retain fluid well. During hot days, not consuming an appropriate amount of water leads to decreased cardiac output and increased body temperature. Elderly people who become dehydrated on a hot day are especially likely to collapse from heat exhaustion.

Other elderly patients may be confined to a bed and unable to access sufficient water, becoming dehydrated. It is important that bedridden patients are carefully supervised and have adequate access to water.

Exercise is a centerpiece to remaining fit but requires the delivery of oxygen and nutrients to the muscles and the regulation and dissipation of body heat. If the heart is not fit enough to handle a level of exercise that varies depending on one's physical shape, the patient can collapse. The decision to start an exercise program should be accompanied by a medical evaluation to determine the fitness level. During exercise, fluid intake is essential. The heart, blood flow to the skin, and the balance of minerals in the body depend upon fluids [42].

5.6 Conclusion

Nonmechanical falls are associated with inherent health problems. Patients should be screened for falls, and if they are unsteady, frightful of a fall, or have a recent history of falls, they should undergo an in-depth evaluation to determine the risk of falling and, secondly, the risks of a consequential serious injury. The plan of care depends on the underlying disease, the state of debilitation, and the exact risks. Modifiable risk factors include getting vision checked, ensuring proper footwear, proper nutrition, and exercising to improve balance and strength.

References

1. Gillespie LD, Gillespie WJ, Robertson MC, Lamb SE, Cumming RG, Rowe BH. Interventions for preventing falls in elderly people. Cochrane Database Syst Rev. 2001;3:Cd000340. https://doi.org/10.1002/14651858.Cd000340.

References

2. Cadore EL, Rodríguez-Mañas L, Sinclair A, Izquierdo M. Effects of different exercise interventions on risk of falls, gait ability, and balance in physically frail older adults: a systematic review. Rejuvenation Res. 2013;16(2):105–14. https://doi.org/10.1089/rej.2012.1397.
3. Yamada M, Arai H, Sonoda T, Aoyama T. Community-based exercise program is cost-effective by preventing care and disability in Japanese frail older adults. J Am Med Dir Assoc. 2012;13(6):507–11. https://doi.org/10.1016/j.jamda.2012.04.001.
4. Robertson MC, Campbell AJ, Gardner MM, Devlin N. Preventing injuries in older people by preventing falls: a meta-analysis of individual-level data. J Am Geriatr Soc. 2002;50(5):905–11. https://doi.org/10.1046/j.1532-5415.2002.50218.x.
5. Lewis CE, Fine LJ, Beddhu S, Cheung AK, Cushman WC, Cutler JA, et al. Final report of a trial of intensive versus standard blood-pressure control. N Engl J Med. 2021;384(20):1921–30. https://doi.org/10.1056/NEJMoa1901281.
6. Rapp SR, Gaussoin SA, Sachs BC, Chelune G, Supiano MA, Lerner AJ, et al. Effects of intensive versus standard blood pressure control on domain-specific cognitive function: a substudy of the SPRINT randomised controlled trial. Lancet Neurol. 2020;19(11):899–907. https://doi.org/10.1016/s1474-4422(20)30319-7.
7. Akinapelli A, Bansal O, Chen JP, Pflugfelder A, Gordon N, Stein K, et al. Left atrial appendage closure -the WATCHMAN device. Curr Cardiol Rev. 2015;11(4):334–40. https://doi.org/10.2174/1573403x11666150805115822.
8. Pang MY, Eng JJ. Muscle strength is a determinant of bone mineral content in the hemiparetic upper extremity: implications for stroke rehabilitation. Bone. 2005;37(1):103–11. https://doi.org/10.1016/j.bone.2005.03.009.
9. Pang MY, Eng JJ, Dawson AS, McKay HA, Harris JE. A community-based fitness and mobility exercise program for older adults with chronic stroke: a randomized, controlled trial. J Am Geriatr Soc. 2005;53(10):1667–74. https://doi.org/10.1111/j.1532-5415.2005.53521.x.
10. Pang MY, Eng JJ, McKay HA, Dawson AS. Reduced hip bone mineral density is related to physical fitness and leg lean mass in ambulatory individuals with chronic stroke. Osteoporos Int. 2005;16(12):1769–79. https://doi.org/10.1007/s00198-005-1925-1.
11. Pang MY, Eng JJ, Dawson AS. Relationship between ambulatory capacity and cardio-respiratory fitness in chronic stroke: influence of stroke-specific impairments. Chest. 2005;127(2):495–501. https://doi.org/10.1378/chest.127.2.495.
12. Eng JJ. Fitness and mobility exercise (FAME) program for stroke. Top Geriatr Rehabil. 2010;26(4):310–23. https://doi.org/10.1097/TGR.0b013e3181fee736.
13. van Poelgeest EP, Pronk AC, Rhebergen D, van der Velde N. Depression, antidepressants and fall risk: therapeutic dilemmas-a clinical review. Eur Geriatr Med. 2021;12(3):585–96. https://doi.org/10.1007/s41999-021-00475-7.
14. Seppala LJ, Petrovic M, Ryg J, Bahat G, Topinkova E, Szczerbińska K, et al. STOPPFall (screening tool of older persons prescriptions in older adults with high fall risk): a Delphi study by the EuGMS task and finish group on fall-risk-increasing drugs. Age Ageing. 2020;50(4):1189–99. https://doi.org/10.1093/ageing/afaa249.
15. Kutner NG, Zhang R, Huang Y, Wasse H. Falls among hemodialysis patients: potential opportunities for prevention? Clin Kidney J. 2014;7(3):257–63. https://doi.org/10.1093/ckj/sfu034.
16. López-Soto PJ, De Giorgi A, Senno E, Tiseo R, Ferraresi A, Canella C, et al. Renal disease and accidental falls: a review of published evidence. BMC Nephrol. 2015;16:176. https://doi.org/10.1186/s12882-015-0173-7.
17. Angalakuditi MV, Gomes J, Coley KC. Impact of drug use and comorbidities on in-hospital falls in patients with chronic kidney disease. Ann Pharmacother. 2007;41(10):1638–43. https://doi.org/10.1345/aph.1H631.
18. Flythe JE, Kimmel SE, Brunelli SM. Rapid fluid removal during dialysis is associated with cardiovascular morbidity and mortality. Kidney Int. 2011;79(2):250–7. https://doi.org/10.1038/ki.2010.383.
19. Zhang W, Zhang S, Deng Y, Wu S, Ren J, Sun G, et al. Trial of intensive blood-pressure control in older patients with hypertension. N Engl J Med. 2021;385(14):1268–79. https://doi.org/10.1056/NEJMoa2111437.

20. Wright JT Jr, Williamson JD, Whelton PK, Snyder JK, Sink KM, Rocco MV, et al. A randomized trial of intensive versus standard blood-pressure control. N Engl J Med. 2015;373(22):2103–16. https://doi.org/10.1056/NEJMoa1511939.
21. Williamson JD, Supiano MA, Applegate WB, Berlowitz DR, Campbell RC, Chertow GM, et al. Intensive vs standard blood pressure control and cardiovascular disease outcomes in adults aged ≥75 years: a randomized clinical trial. JAMA. 2016;315(24):2673–82. https://doi.org/10.1001/jama.2016.7050.
22. Benetos A, Labat C, Rossignol P, Fay R, Rolland Y, Valbusa F, et al. Treatment with multiple blood pressure medications, achieved blood pressure, and mortality in older nursing home residents: the PARTAGE study. JAMA Intern Med. 2015;175(6):989–95. https://doi.org/10.1001/jamainternmed.2014.8012.
23. Shimbo D, Barrett Bowling C, Levitan EB, Deng L, Sim JJ, Huang L, et al. Short-term risk of serious fall injuries in older adults initiating and intensifying treatment with antihypertensive medication. Circ Cardiovasc Qual Outcomes. 2016;9(3):222–9. https://doi.org/10.1161/circoutcomes.115.002524.
24. Butt DA, Mamdani M, Austin PC, Tu K, Gomes T, Glazier RH. The risk of hip fracture after initiating antihypertensive drugs in the elderly. Arch Intern Med. 2012;172(22):1739–44. https://doi.org/10.1001/2013.jamainternmed.469.
25. Rivasi G, Ceolin L, Capacci M, Matteucci G, Testa GD, Ungar A. Risks associated with intensive blood pressure control in older patients. Kardiol Pol. 2023; https://doi.org/10.33963/KP.a2022.0297.
26. Oh M, Ylitalo KR. Joint Association of diabetes and physical activity with falls among midlife and older adults: 2018 behavioral risk factor surveillance system. Am J Health Promot. 2022:8901171221141077. https://doi.org/10.1177/08901171221141077.
27. Joseph A, Wanono R, Flamant M, Vidal-Petiot E. Orthostatic hypotension: a review. Nephrol Ther. 2017;13(Suppl 1):S55–s67. https://doi.org/10.1016/j.nephro.2017.01.003.
28. Lin CK, Lin CC. Work of breathing and respiratory drive in obesity. Respirology. 2012;17(3):402–11. https://doi.org/10.1111/j.1440-1843.2011.02124.x.
29. Zumrutbas AE, Bozkurt AI, Alkis O, Toktas C, Cetinel B, Aybek Z. The prevalence of nocturia and nocturnal polyuria: can new cutoff values be suggested according to age and sex? Int Neurourol J. 2016;20(4):304–10. https://doi.org/10.5213/inj.1632558.279.
30. Pesonen JS, Vernooij RWM, Cartwright R, Aoki Y, Agarwal A, Mangera A, et al. The impact of nocturia on falls and fractures: a systematic review and meta-analysis. J Urol. 2020;203(4):674–83. https://doi.org/10.1097/JU.0000000000000459.
31. Shakoor N, Furmanov S, Nelson DE, Li Y, Block JA. Pain and its relationship with muscle strength and proprioception in knee OA: results of an 8-week home exercise pilot study. J Musculoskelet Neuronal Interact. 2008;8(1):35–42.
32. Gordt K, Gerhardy T, Najafi B, Schwenk M. Effects of wearable sensor-based balance and gait training on balance, gait, and functional performance in healthy and patient populations: a systematic review and meta-analysis of randomized controlled trials. Gerontology. 2017;64(1):74–89. https://doi.org/10.1159/000481454.
33. Alfieri A, Martone D, Randers MB, Labruna G, Mancini A, Nielsen JJ, et al. Effects of long-term football training on the expression profile of genes involved in muscle oxidative metabolism. Mol Cell Probes. 2015;29(1):43–7. https://doi.org/10.1016/j.mcp.2014.11.003.
34. Krustrup P, Williams CA, Mohr M, Hansen PR, Helge EW, Elbe AM, et al. The "football is medicine" platform-scientific evidence, large-scale implementation of evidence-based concepts and future perspectives. Scand J Med Sci Sports. 2018;28(Suppl 1):3–7. https://doi.org/10.1111/sms.13220.
35. Semenova EA, Pranckevičienė E, Bondareva EA, Gabdrakhmanova LJ, Ahmetov II. Identification and characterization of genomic predictors of sarcopenia and sarcopenic obesity using UK biobank data. Nutrients. 2023;15(3) https://doi.org/10.3390/nu15030758.

References

36. Tofthagen C, Visovsky C, Berry DL. Strength and balance training for adults with peripheral neuropathy and high risk of fall: current evidence and implications for future research. Oncol Nurs Forum. 2012;39(5):E416–24. https://doi.org/10.1188/12.Onf.E416-e424.
37. Wylie G, Torrens C, Campbell P, Frost H, Gordon AL, Menz HB, et al. Podiatry interventions to prevent falls in older people: a systematic review and meta-analysis. Age Ageing. 2019;48(3):327–36. https://doi.org/10.1093/ageing/afy189.
38. Wylie G, Menz HB, McFarlane S, Ogston S, Sullivan F, Williams B, et al. Podiatry intervention versus usual care to prevent falls in care homes: pilot randomised controlled trial (the PIRFECT study). BMC Geriatr. 2017;17(1):143. https://doi.org/10.1186/s12877-017-0541-1.
39. LeBoff MS, Greenspan SL, Insogna KL, Lewiecki EM, Saag KG, Singer AJ, et al. The clinician's guide to prevention and treatment of osteoporosis. Osteoporos Int. 2022;33(10):2049–102. https://doi.org/10.1007/s00198-021-05900-y.
40. Chomistek AK, Chiuve SE, Jensen MK, Cook NR, Rimm EB. Vigorous physical activity, mediating biomarkers, and risk of myocardial infarction. Med Sci Sports Exerc. 2011;43(10):1884–90. https://doi.org/10.1249/MSS.0b013e31821b4d0a.
41. Hamrick I, Norton D, Birstler J, Chen G, Cruz L, Hanrahan L. Association between dehydration and falls. Mayo Clin Proc Innov Qual Outcomes. 2020;4(3):259–65. https://doi.org/10.1016/j.mayocpiqo.2020.01.003.
42. Wingo JE. Exercise intensity prescription during heat stress: a brief review. Scand J Med Sci Sports. 2015;25(Suppl 1):90–5. https://doi.org/10.1111/sms.12381.

Chapter 6
Preventing Mechanical Falls

6.1 Introduction

Mechanical falls are generally unexpected. Patients who fall often say they tripped over a step or slipped on some water. While these are environmental and potentially avoidable, an underlying medical disorder often contributes to the fall. For this reason, efforts should be made to anticipate and remove potential fall obstacles that can injure a person known to be a fall risk. This chapter aims to identify ways to remove the hazard along the site where a loved one, a friend, a patient, or even you could fall. Falls can result from a composite of events, and proactively identifying and eliminating these circumstances can reduce the chance of an injurious fall. Table 6.1 is based on the Table 6.1 of Chap. 3. In Chap. 3, the major causes of mechanical falls were presented. Discovering the cause is the major step in solving the problem. In this chapter, the focus will be solely on how falls for each of these topics can be prevented.

6.2 Home

The common theme throughout this chapter is that proper planning is key in preventing accidents in persons with fall risks. This planning and construction optimally occur before the resident occupies the properly. Many codes and guidelines are available, and it is time well spent for prospective owners and their contractors to carefully orchestrate these concepts in order to create a safe environment for the vulnerable.

Table 6.1 Measures to prevent falls

HOME
1. Handrails
2. Keeping surfaces dry
3. Using bath mats and grab bars
4. Avoiding uneven surfaces and jutting edges
5. Keeping rugs and carpets wrinkle-free
6. Using ladders safely
7. Avoiding clutter
8. Night-lights
9. Assistive devices
10. Wheelchairs
11. Standing slowly
OUTDOORS
1. Using walking sticks
2. Footwear for hiking
3. The hat
4. Sunscreen
5. Staying hydrated
6. Headlamps
7. Avoiding dangers

6.2.1 Handrails

Losing balance and falling on stairs is the second most common cause of injury in persons over age 65. Approximately one million stair injuries that require emergency care occur each year.

Falls downstairs are common causes of foot or ankle fractures and shoulder injuries. The risk of a lower extremity fracture from a staircase accident is doubled that of one standing still. About 21.6% of stair-related injuries involve the head and neck [1]. Gait instability, a common occurrence that accompanies aging, contributes to falls on stairs. A slippery surface can cause one to lose balance, and holding on to the rail (as one should be) could also contribute to a rotator cuff injury.

Stairs should have handrails on both sides. They should be well lit and have a nonstick surface on the steps. Thick carpeting on the stairs may induce falls. The stairs should be free of clutter and should not be worn, damaged, or slippery.

A common mistake when going up or down the stairs while shopping is to try to carry purchases upstairs using both hands and not holding on to the handrail. In the movie theater, carrying popcorn and a soft drink up the stairs with both hands can be treacherous. When there is only one point of contact with the stairs, an unsteady foot in those prone to instability or gait disturbances invites trouble. Additionally, the view of the stairs and the path ahead may be blocked by the object one carries. It is far better to use the elevator or carry fewer items and make an extra trip.

6.2 Home

A fall on the stairs can happen if one slips, losing footing. Stairways have a prescribed width that is established by international residential codes. They should not be less than 36 inches and, with handrails, 27 inches across. The headroom should be at least 6 feet 8 inches. Stairs cannot be continuous and must have a break at 151 inches. The stair must not rise under 7 ¾ inches, The tread depth should be 11 inches minimum. The handrail height should be between 34 and 38 inches. International building codes can be found on the web at **https://codes.iccsafe.org/**.

When traveling, the elderly should be very cautious. Although some notable buildings, like the back entrance to the US Capitol (Fig. 6.1), do have handrails, many famous buildings and monuments that may be on your "bucket list" do not have handrails (see Fig. 6.2). One's personal safety should guide the decision to visit them. A serious fall will ruin what was intended to be an enjoyable day.

6.2.2 Keeping Surfaces Dry

A slippery surface increases the risk of a fall for a vulnerable individual. This is, to some extent, preventable from a planning perspective by using ceramics or flooring that has a high dynamic coefficient of friction (DCOF). This value is the rating on

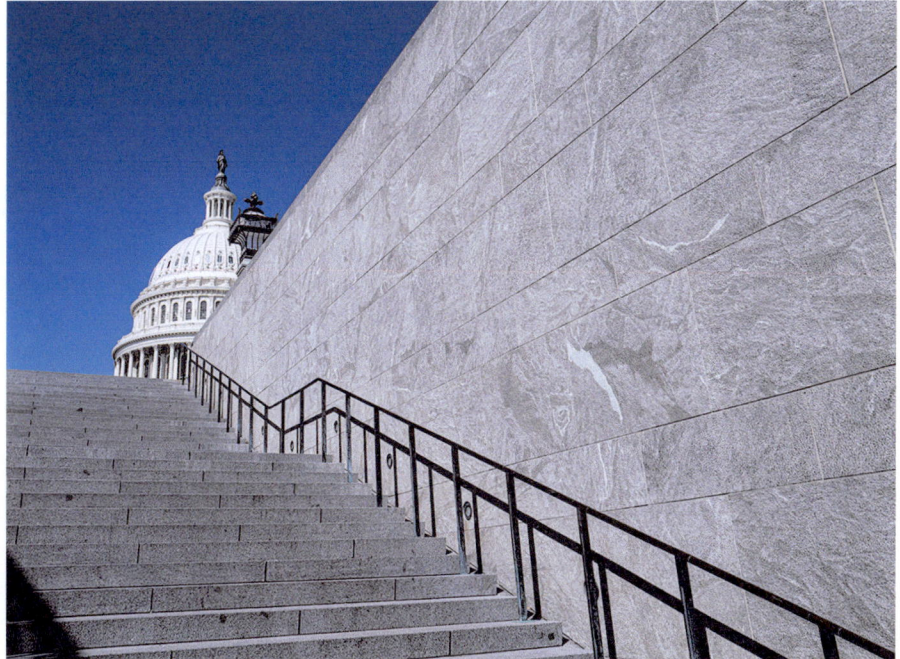

Fig. 6.1 Handrails prevent falls. Trying to walk on the stairs while holding objects and not holding on to the rails is a fall risk, particularly in the elderly. Photo by Stephen Fadem

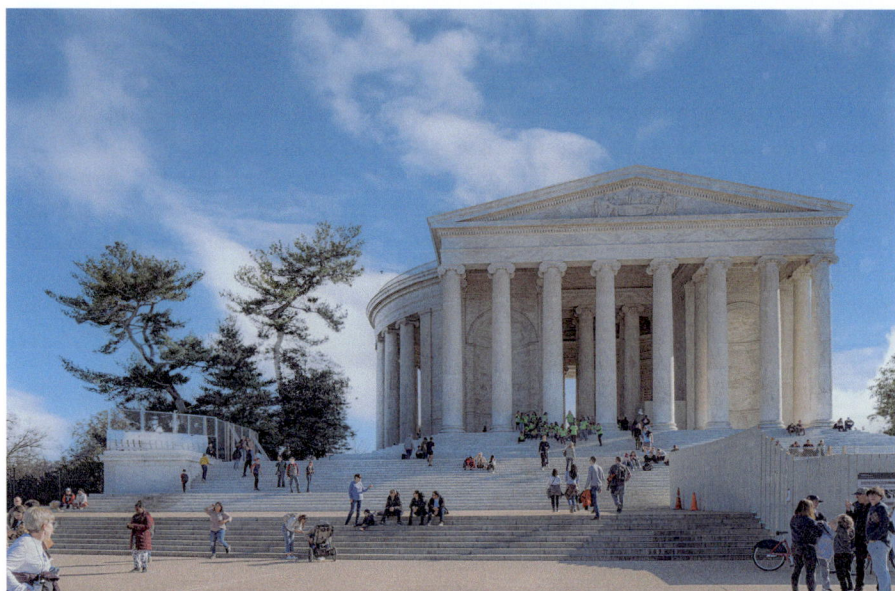

Fig. 6.2 The Jefferson Memorial is a beautiful structure done in the classical style. Handrails are not apparent, but the building is being renovated. Photo by Stephen Fadem

surface flooring that determines its slickness property. If the DCOF is <0.4, it is considered very slippery. A DCOF less than 0.42 is considered slippery when wet, and balconies, ramps, wheelchair ramps, and sidewalks are required to have a DCOF ≥0.65. (**https://tcnatile.com/**). Regardless, the surface must be kept clean and free of any slippery fluids like oil, other liquids, and water. Any spills should be wiped up immediately. The floor should be cleaned according to the manufacturer's instructions and not over-waxed. Antislip footwear should be worn. The use of stockings or any footwear without traction is not advisable. Areas where the vulnerable may walk should be clean, dry, and clutter-free. Those who are unstable should take their time when walking on a potentially slippery surface and may require an assistive device or personal assistance. Ramps should have handrails, and all areas should be well-lit.

Special soles on footwear have been designed to walk on ice and other slippery surfaces (see Fig. 6.3). These items are readily available in sporting goods stores.

6.2.3 Using Bath Mats and Grab Bars

Falling backward while attempting to get out of the bathtub is the most common cause of death from falls. Bathing in hot water dilates the blood vessels and redistributes the body's blood volume. This can drop blood pressure such that dizziness

6.2 Home

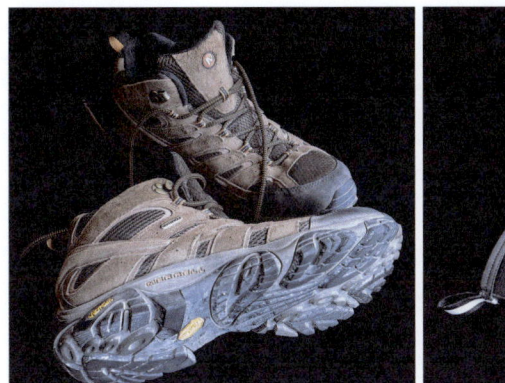 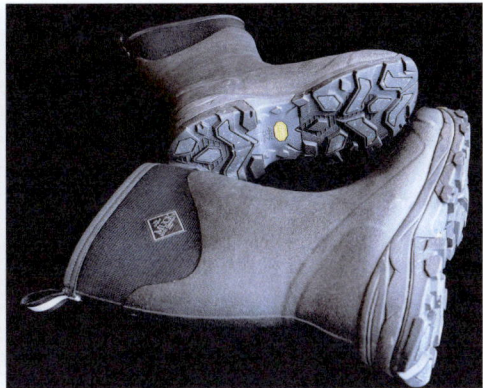

Fig. 6.3 Soles designed to address slippery surfaces, even ice

and loss of balance can occur when one suddenly stands. Bath seats can be helpful, so can grab bars. One must get up slowly, and if dizziness starts, sit back down immediately. Having the smartphone on the nearby dressing table can help since Siri and Google can either call emergency services, your loved one, or your provider. People with grab bars recover their balance 75.8% more often than those who do not have them. This is the most successful environmental strategy to protect against a fall. They are recommended to support bathing tasks and have been validated to be helpful [2]. Having a bench in the bathtub or shower will allow one to sit down quickly if feeling like passing out.

Many hotels are using walk-in showers rather than tubs. These have advantages in that one does not have the chance to stand up in a pool of hot water after bathing. The showers have grab bars and handheld washing devices for safety and convenience (Fig. 6.4).

When falling, many patients will grab the towel bar or sink edge. Replacing the towel bars with grab bars and using nonslip adhesive strips on the sink edge can prevent slippage. The toilet seat should be elevated if the resident is wheelchair-bound. Figure 6.5 shows an ideal way to use grab bars in the toilet area.

Grab bars come in a variety of configurations. The Americans with Disabilities Act (ADA) website has authored guidelines covering bathroom design standards (**https://www.ada.gov/law-and-regs/design-standards/standards-guidance/**).

6.2.4 *Avoiding Uneven Surfaces and Jutting Edges*

Uneven surfaces and small steps can surprise an elderly person with mobility issues, causing one to lose balance and fall. It is easy to become distracted when walking since ambulating is such an everyday part of our routine. Combine inattentiveness, an uneven surface, and a gait disorder, and there is a setup for a fall. Gravel, snow,

Fig. 6.4 Grab bars in a walk-in shower

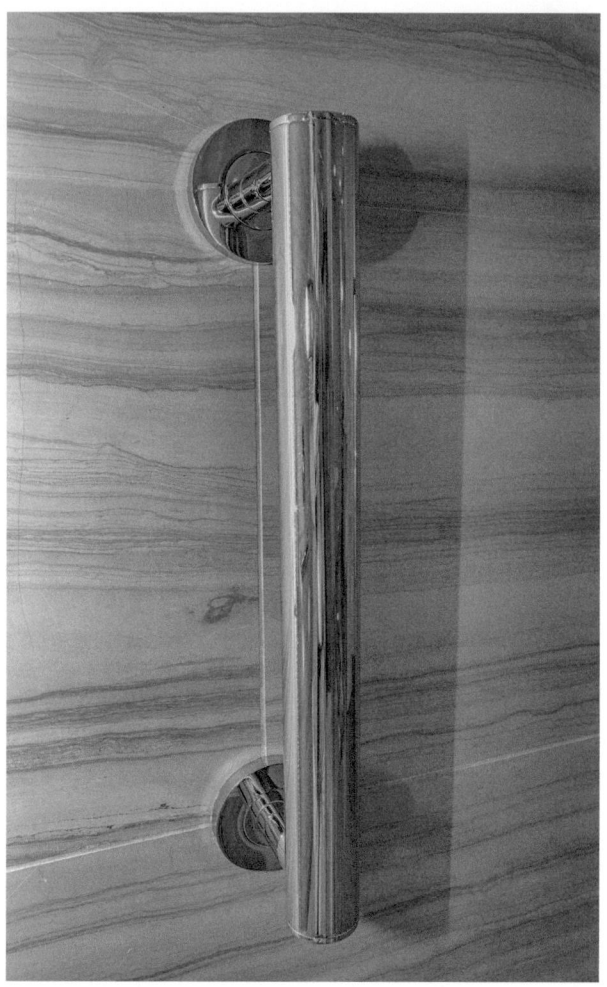

ice, leaves, and uneven pavement cause 19 times as many serious injuries as collision road accidents [3]. Parking blocks can also cause falls (see Fig. 6.6). The most common injury from a fall while walking is a fracture. The fracture results from a direct hit on an outstretched hand, the femoral neck (hip), or the ankle [4]. The fall occurs if the person cannot regain balance using a recovery step and is carried to the ground by forward momentum. Although it is not always possible to prevent this type of fall, training and exercises can strengthen bones and muscles and help people develop muscle memory for recovery. If a fall is imminent, it is possible to lean into it, protect the head, and try to land on a safe and cushioned part of the body. Bump hats are inexpensive and resemble the popular baseball cap. They contain a plastic lining, helping to soften the blow and reduce the possibility of a head injury. Padded workout clothes also are readily available online. They may help prevent a hip injury.

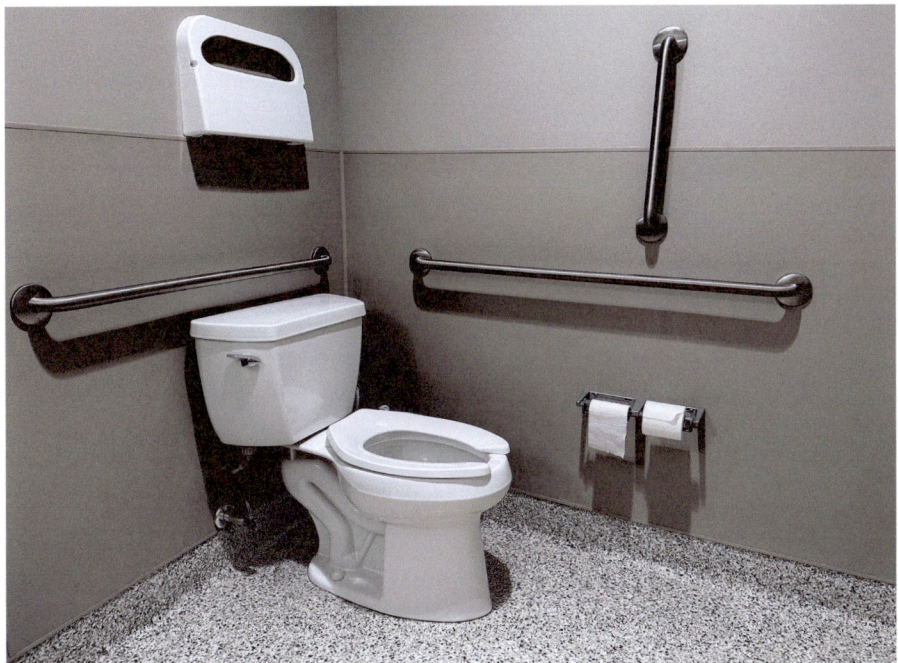

Fig. 6.5 Grab bars placement in a public bathroom

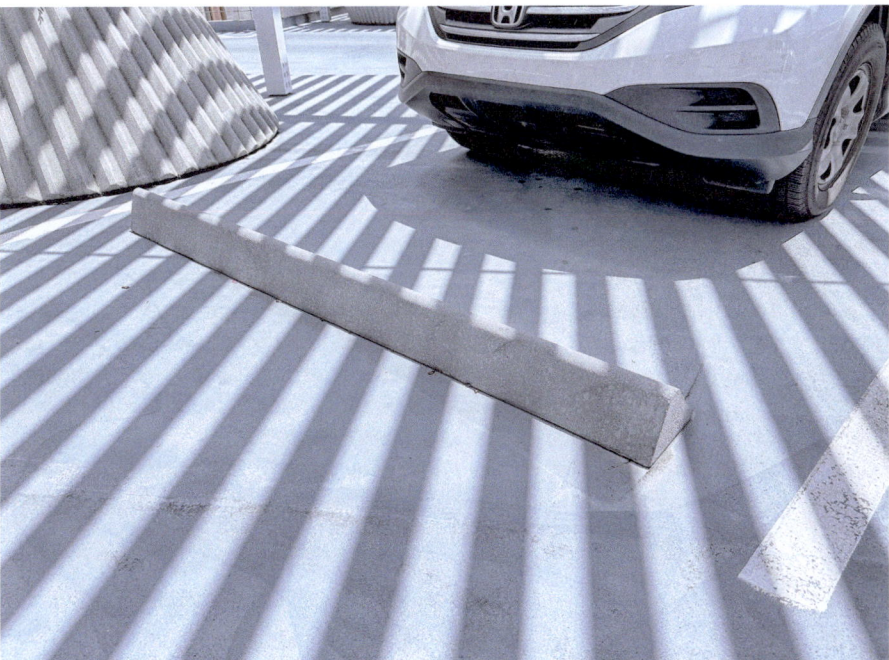

Fig. 6.6 It is easy to trip over uneven surfaces or parking blocks. Those with impairments should use caution and be aware of this potential hazard

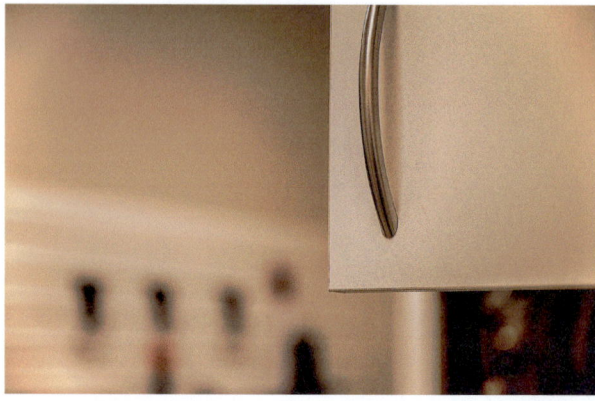

Fig. 6.7 Jutting objects like cabinet doors can cause substantial injuries. Low-hanging tree branches can also cause head trauma

The bump hat may be especially useful when preventing an injury from jutting objects. Tree branches and cabinet doors that have been left open are hazards because a person can accidentally hit their head against them (see Fig. 6.7) . Potential injuries include trauma to the eye or face, a concussion, or even significant brain injury. Prevention begins with never leaving cabinet doors open. One must be mindful when walking and pay attention to the surroundings as much as possible. Hiking in groups will help to minimize the dangers of jutting tree branches.

6.2.5 Keeping Rugs and Carpets Wrinkle Free

If wall-to-wall carpets or small-area rugs are not secured, they can easily move when walked on, throwing one off balance (see Fig. 6.8). Uneven, wrinkled, and worn carpets are a common cause of accidents. Rugs should be secured with a nonslip pad. Women tend to fall more than men, but men sustain a higher incidence of head, neck, and traumatic brain injuries. Many injuries occur when hastily transitioning from surface to surface. Proactively straighten rugs and repair damaged and worn areas. Avoiding hurrying and increasing awareness of this type of hazard will help. Rugs and carpets should be secured with adhesive tape or strong backing material. Environmental modifications should be accompanied by fall prevention strategies that include vision checks, medication reviews, assessments of gait and balance by occupational therapists, and exercise to improve balance and muscle strength. The use of vitamin D, bone-building exercises, and the avoidance of inactivity and metabolic acidosis can help maintain bones [5].

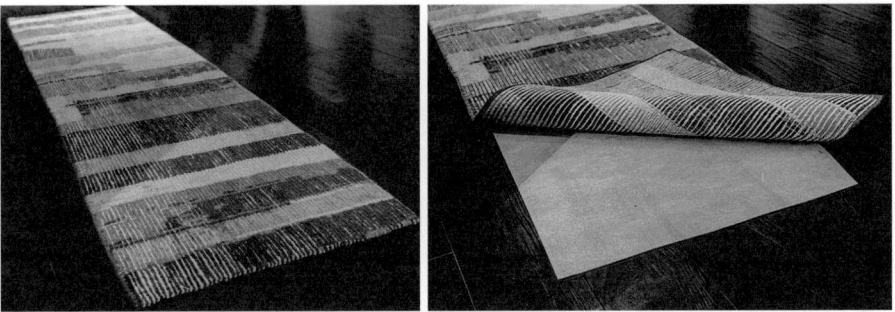

Fig. 6.8 Securing a rug with padding and keeping it wrinkle free helps prevent falls

6.2.6 Using Ladders Safely

Ladder accidents are dangerous and cause fatal falls in elderly people (see Fig. 6.9). With impaired balance, it is best to rely on a friend, handyman, younger loved one, or neighbor to grab the out-of-reach items and change lightbulbs. Ensure the ladder is not damaged, missing rungs, bolts, cleats, screws, or any other component. Damaged ladders should be appropriately marked "Do not use." Ladder-related accidents can be decreased with proper training. If climbing a ladder, always hold on with one hand, ensure the ladder is opened and set up properly, secure, and steady, and have someone accompany you. Accidents occur when one does not hold on or loses footing. Never step above the second-highest step on the step ladder. It is best to avoid extension ladders unless you are experienced with ladder use, have undergone ladder safety training, are familiar with the National Institute for Occupational Safety & Health (NIOSH)'s NIOSH angle measuring tool, and have no recently diagnosed balance or gait disorders. If finding yourself the least bit shaky while starting to climb, get back down! Nothing you are going to do on top of a ladder is so urgent it necessitates an ambulance ride to the emergency room with a traumatic brain injury or a fractured cervical spine (broken neck) (**https://www.cdc.gov/niosh/newsroom/feature/ladder-safety.html**).

Instead of a ladder, using a slim, lightweight, inexpensive grabber might be safer. This invaluable device can be purchased for less than $13.00 USD (Fig. 6.10).

6.2.7 Avoiding Clutter

Half of all falls occur because of tripping over an object left on the floor (Fig. 6.11). If one makes an impact with an object, the change in the swing motion sets up a loss of balance. There are several ways to prevent tripping over clutter, but many require being proactive. Having hooks, shelves, and designated places that are off-path, can help create a habit of hanging up clothing or quickly folding it and placing it on a

Fig. 6.9 Ladders at either home or the workplace should be set up appropriately to avoid malfunction and secondary injury

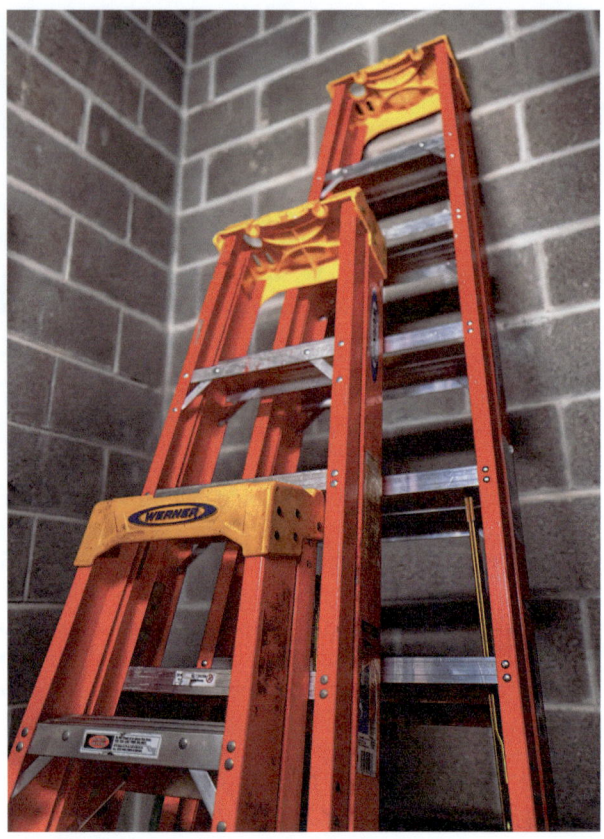

Fig. 6.10 Grabbers are inexpensive and useful for getting objects that are out of reach

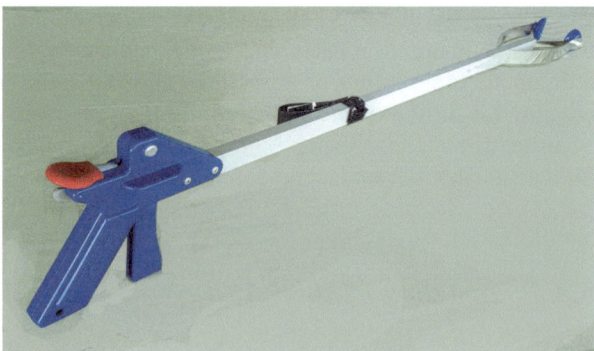

6.2 Home

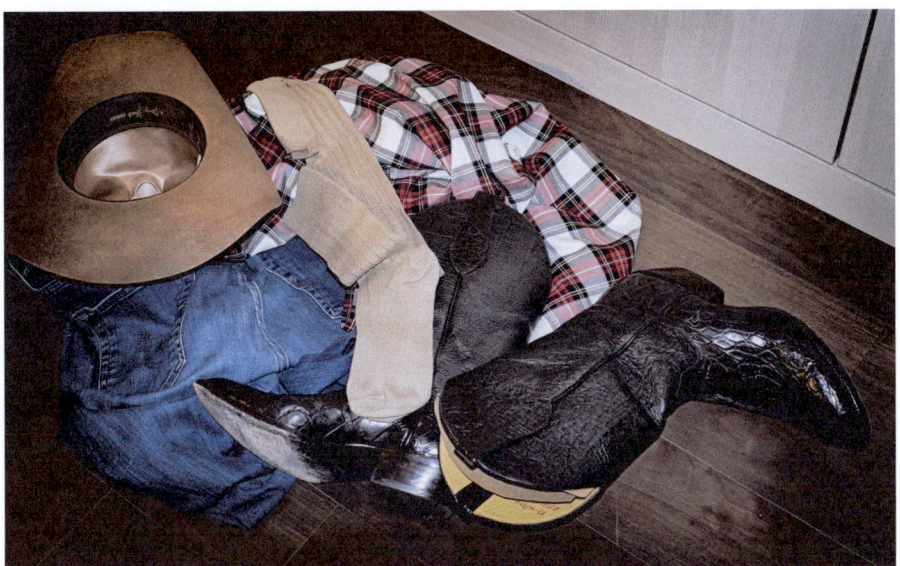

Fig. 6.11 While a young cowboy probably will not get hurt tripping over cluttered clothing, an older individual may be at risk

shelf. Ensure the path is well-lit. Proper footwear can help support balance. Training and exercise can help build balance and muscle and bone strength. Practicing recovery steps and ensuring upper leg strength can support a sudden balance shift may help prevent a fall or lessen the injury. Look for alternate outlets so that wires and cords that are strung across the floor (see Fig. 6.12). Furniture placement is important; ensure that it does not partially occlude the pathway. Tripping can also occur when using an assistive device such as a walker.

6.2.8 Night-Lights

Vision is one of the senses that feeds into balance control, integrating signals from the inner ear, joints and muscles, and eyes. In the dark, it may be harder to maintain balance. Furthermore, it is easy to stumble or trip with poor lighting. Night-lights are essential in preventing falls as the sense of balance declines. Night-lights are more effective when placed in the front rather than the back of the path (or both sites) (Fig. 6.13).

Fig. 6.12 A cord lying across the floor is a trip hazard

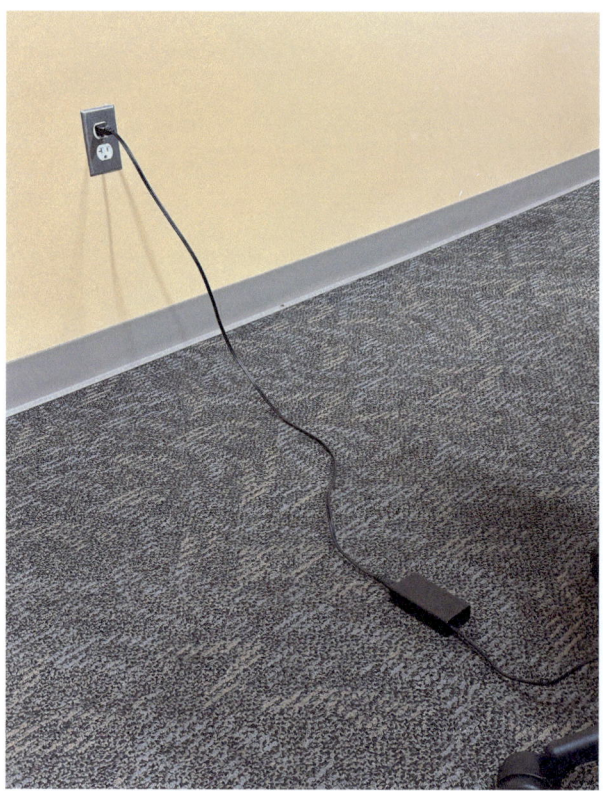

6.2.9 Assistive Devices

Persons with disabilities' problems often require an assistive device. The most commonly used device is a cane, but walkers and rollators are also helpful in preventing falls [6]. Some persons do not use assistive devices because they feel it compromises self-esteem. Feelings like this need to be considered by caregivers. Having an assistive device not only can prevent a fall but can increase mobility and independence.

Proper training is essential when using an assistive device. When improperly used or poorly maintained, an assistive device can contribute to rather than prevent a fall. Device critical component failures, unintended device movement, unable to handle over uneven surfaces, instability (wobbly and insecure), and trip hazards are common pathways to injury. Many injuries can be prevented through the early education and training of both the caregiver and patient. Brakes need to be inspected, tested, and repaired regularly. Poor wheel traction places older adults at risk of falling. Many assistive devices break easily or have loose parts. Half the injuries occur because of component breakage, and better inspection programs are needed to ensure these products' ongoing maintenance and safety. Trip hazard rates are highest with walkers and rollators, associated with seven times the injury rate as canes.

Fig. 6.13 Night-lights are inexpensive and can reduce the risk of a fall

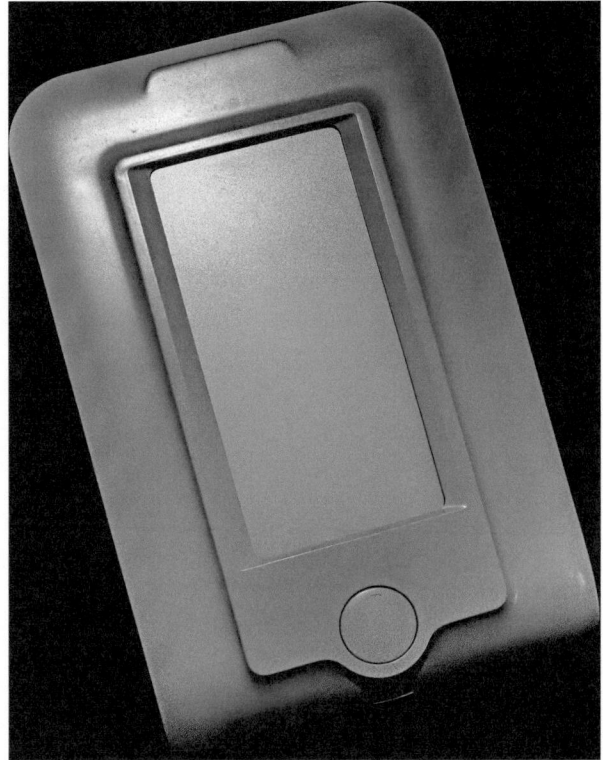

This is due to the balance between stability and ease of use. This may constitute a design failure. Canes with large bases were associated with higher accident rates, as they generate more instability than traditional canes [7].

The use of a standard cane is practical for persons who need support when walking, but canes should not be used for weight-bearing. Walkers should be used when people have muscle weakness or poor balance. Walkers with wheels allow the forward gait stepping to continue but are not as stable as they can unintentionally move. The four-wheeled walker or rollator may not be steady for persons with poor balance. One must have good cognitive function to use a rollator [8].

Assistive devices are useful in preventing falls when properly used. This includes proper training, frequent inspection, and feedback to the manufacturers to improve their design (see Fig. 6.14).

6.2.10 Wheelchairs

About 80.9% of wheelchair accidents because of a trip and fall. Wheelchair training and safety are necessary to prevent this. Wheelchairs should be inspected and maintained, and the wheelchair path should be clear of any environmental hazards.

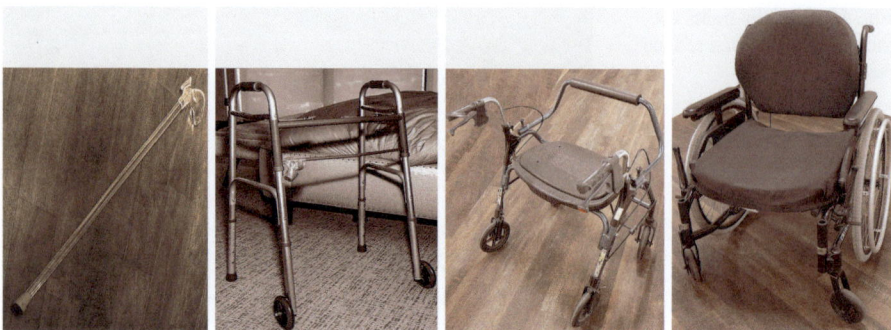

Fig. 6.14 Assistive devices – cane, walker, rollator, wheelchair

Patients and caregivers need to understand braking techniques. About 12.2% of accidents happened during transfers. These generally will happen if the brake is not properly placed. Wheelchair transfer techniques should be learned and practiced by caregivers. Here is the wheelchair transfer guides by the National Institute of Health used for transferring to a dental chair. Transfer principles are similar regardless of where the transfer site is. https://www.nidcr.nih.gov/sites/default/files/2017-09/wheelchair-transfer-provider-guide.pdf [8] (see Fig. 6.14).

6.2.11 Stand Slowly

The blood pressure can easily fall when standing too rapidly for persons with advanced diabetes who have a disorder in how their nervous system regulates blood pressure. Blood pressure medications and dehydration can cause lightheadedness, fainting, or a fall. This is preventable by avoiding a rapid change in position and maintaining adequate hydration. Patients who take blood pressure medications should have their blood pressure and therapy closely monitored [9].

6.3 Outdoors

Falls are a potential hazard to walkers, whether in a national park or in the neighborhood. Certain principles guide safe practices and keep walkers out of trouble. Communication is essential. Hikers in large parks and wilderness areas should never hike alone. Since getting in touch with emergency services may be impossible in areas that are not equipped for cell phone usage, renting a satellite phone should be part of the planning. Satellite phones require a sky view since they work on a line of site.

Likewise, seniors hiking in the neighborhood need a charged cell phone and to understand how to reach a friend, loved one, neighbor, or emergency services. A GPS watcher is useful as an emergency tool and can help a loved one find you if you become lost.

Fatigue and exhaustion can be treacherous if one overexerts oneself, especially if not staying hydrated. It is important to use hiking sticks and be aware of the terrain when hiking. The same principles apply to taking a walk in the neighborhood, particularly for the elderly with decreased balance or muscle strength. Planning is important. Wear a hat, sunscreen, and appropriate clothing, and dress in layers. Use footwear with good traction to avoid slipping.

6.3.1 Using Walking Sticks

Although walking sticks do not support one's weight, they help with balance. They are useful if the terrain is rough or there are steep inclines and declines. Hiking sticks are longer but can be collapsed. They are extremely lightweight and can be packed when traveling. The cane may offer stability in the neighborhood for persons with poor balance. It is smaller, is usually light, and generally has a curved handle.

6.3.2 Footwear

Proper footwear is essential whether climbing rocks or climbing stairs. The forces acting on the feet when climbing stairs are 1.2 times the body weight, and when descending, they can be up to 2.6 times the body weight. The ideal shoes should have shock-absorbing properties and should have a nonslip sole [10]. Well-designed shoes have several advantages – they can stretch, offering an ideal fit for patients with edema, hammertoes, or bunions. An orthotic insole can reduce foot problems such as overpronation, plantar fasciitis, and foot pain. The toe box is wide and soft, with ample padding, arch supports, and deep heel padding. They have natural cushioning and a nonslip outsole. The ideal pair of shoes come in multiple widths. Since walking and hiking preserve muscle and bone function, well-designed footwear makes the hike or walk enjoyable, providing a fun way to maintain health. Shoes should fit snugly and securely. Several popular shoe companies specialize in shoes that are very suitable for seniors, and individual needs vary. The local shoe store can offer good advice about the specific characteristics of the shoes you are looking at. If you have a specific foot condition, consult a podiatrist for added reassurance (see Fig. 6.15).

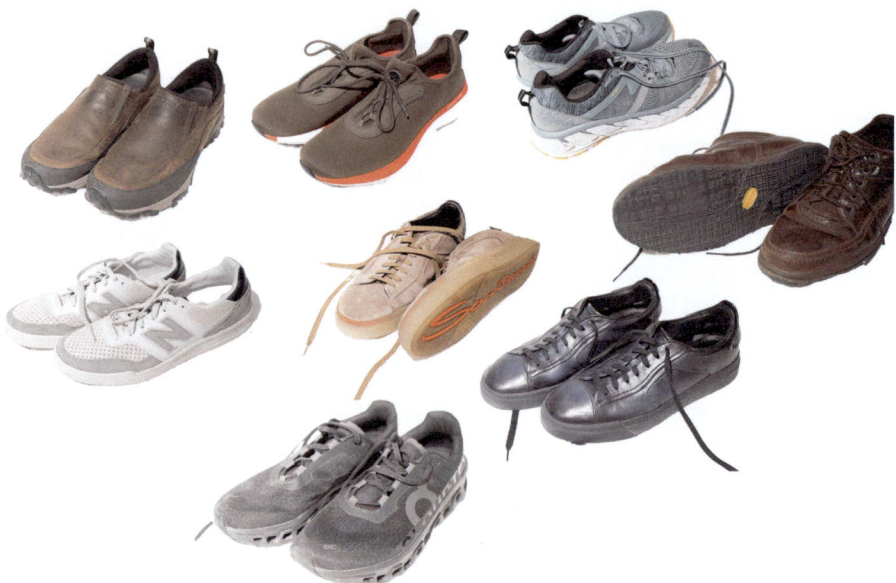

Fig. 6.15 Footwear that has a wide toe box, ample cushioning, good arch support, and a good rubber surface can be purchased in a variety of stores. Special orthopedic and diabetic footwear is also available. Persons with serious gait and foot disorders should be evaluated by a podiatrist

6.3.3 The Hat

Figure 6.16 the wide-brimmed hat protects your head, ears, and face from the sun and keeps you cool. Also, in the event of a fall, the brim may help absorb some of the shocks and help protect your head. Several models of hiking and walking hats are available.

The bump cap offers padded protection and contains a high-density elastic shell. It is not an industrial safety or hard hat and should not be confused with one, as they have different purposes. The protection it offers is limited. Recreational falls comprise 75% of climbing injuries, and head trauma is a common cause of severe injury and death [11]. Hats or helmets may not provide adequate protection and should not be assumed to do so. They are never a substitute for proper planning. The manufacturers recommend that since the plastic deteriorates with time, a bump cap used primarily outdoors be discarded after 2 years and, when used indoors, should be discarded after 5 years (Fig. 6.17).

6.3.4 Sunscreen

While not directly related to fall prevention, wearing sun protection helps prevent skin injury that can lead to squamous cell cancer and melanoma. They work by blocking the short ultraviolet light waves that can cause damage (see Fig. 6.18) [12].

6.3 Outdoors

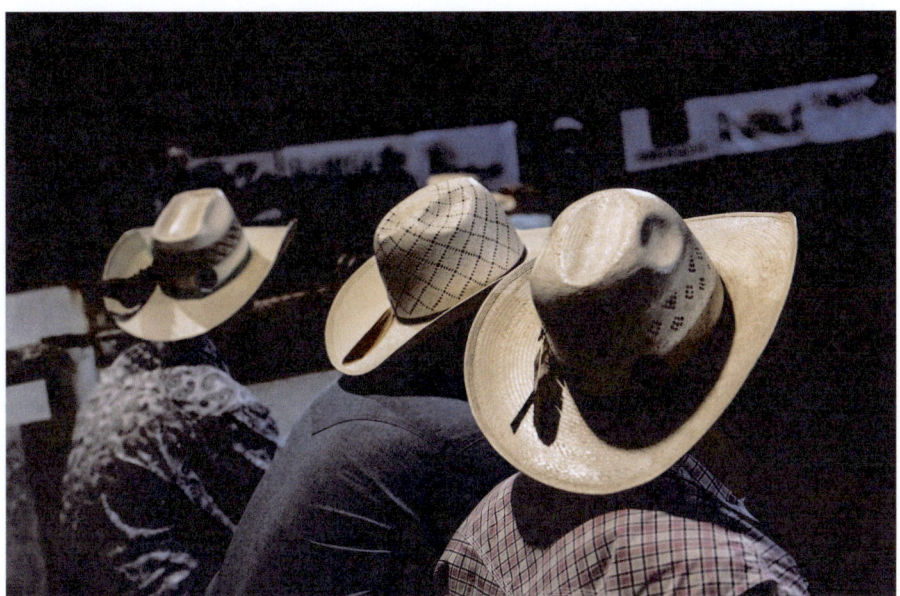

Fig. 6.16 Cowboy hats are one type of protective wide-brim hat

Fig. 6.17 The bump cap costs around $20.00 USD. It can be worn unobtrusively and may help protect from an injury during a fall

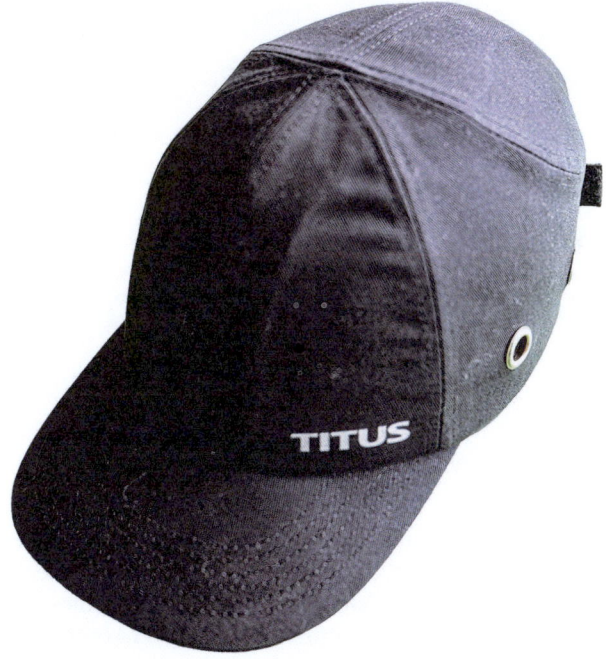

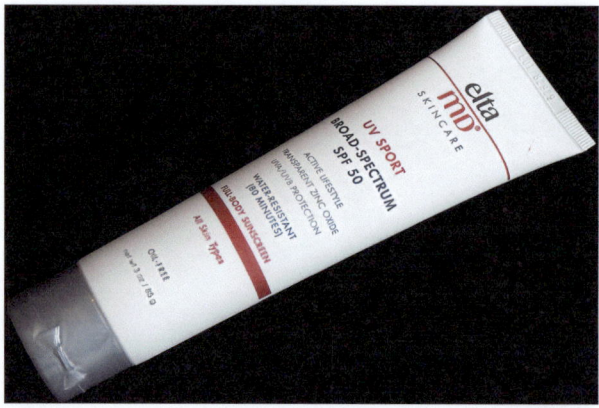

Fig. 6.18 Sun protection might not help prevent a fall but will protect against developing skin cancer. Sunburns can be miserable and are avoidable

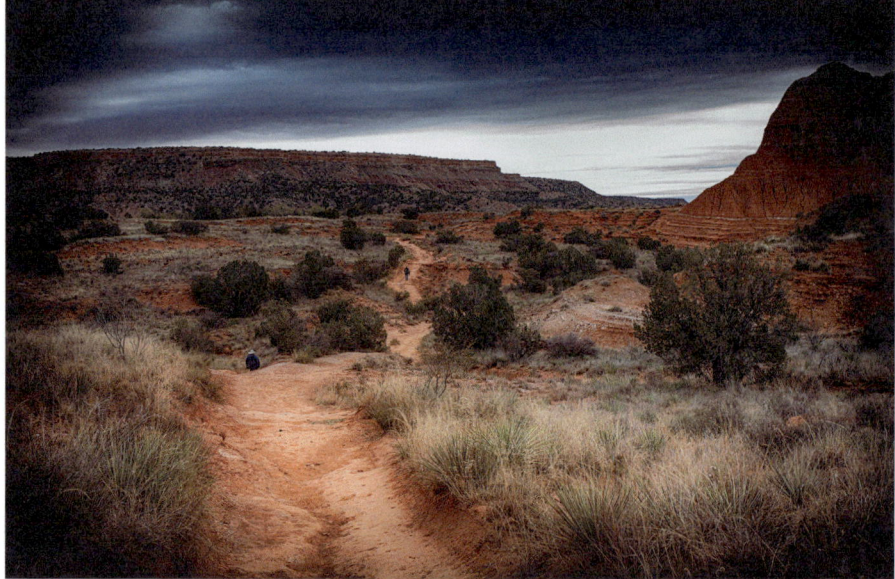

Fig. 6.19 Scene from a trail at Big Bend Ranch State Park. Hike with a buddy, use a walking stick, wear good shoes, and take an ample water supply

6.3.5 Staying Hydrated

Deaths from heat exhaustion are frequent in the Big Bend parks (see Fig. 6.19) This huge region is part of the Chihuahua Desert that extends across the Rio Grande River into Mexico. Generally, the person who dies is an experienced hiker who is out alone. What seems at first like a fun and exciting trail becomes more arduous as time passes. The hiker does not appreciate the extreme weather conditions and does not bring ample water. Sweating is a means of cooling off the body, but it comes

6.3 Outdoors

with a price – loss of fluid reserves that must be replenished. Fluid balance is necessary for the body to function. Hiking or walking without proper water intake can lead to an inability to rid the body of heat. The biochemical reactions that keep us alive work within a limited temperature range, above which we develop exhaustion and heat stroke.

6.3.6 Headlamps

When walking in the dark, wear a headlamp. Using the headlamp in the neighborhood will provide the light to help you maintain your balance and avoid obstacles on the ground. Oncoming cars can also see and avoid you. Headlamps are inexpensive and an invaluable part of either a hike on a trail or a walk in the city.

6.3.7 Avoid Danger

Balanced Rock (Fig. 6.20) is the culmination of the Grapevine Hill trail in Big Bend National Park. It is a short, unfriendly, technical, challenging, steep, quarter-mile climb that takes balance, coordination, and very strong thigh muscles. Medical care in this deserted area is sparse. Getting to the spot where this photo was taken can be

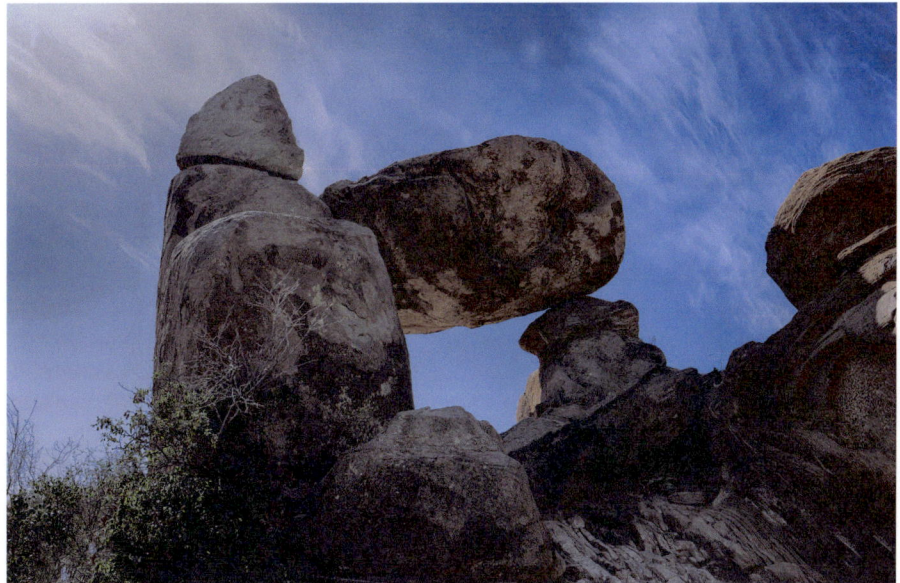

Fig. 6.20 Balanced Rock – Big Bend National Park – Photo by Stephen Fadem

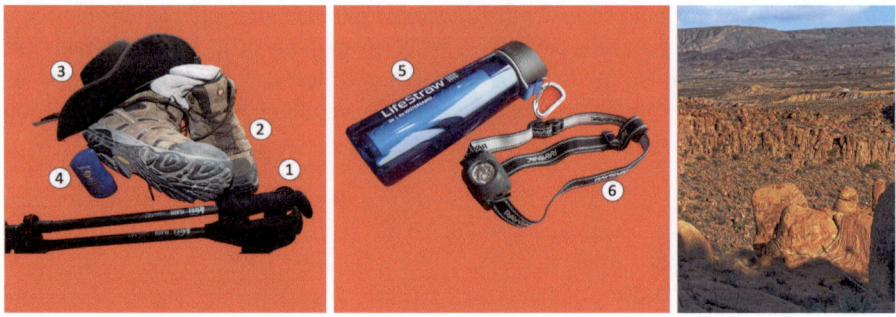

Fig. 6.21 When hiking outdoors use (1) use walking sticks, (2) wear proper footwear, (3) don't forget a hat, (4) put on sunscreen (5) stay hydrated, (6) if hiking to a sunrise or back from a sunset, or stargazing at night, use a headlamp and (7) above all avoid dangerous ledges and technical climbing that is beyond your experience and skill level

exhausting. If not in condition, efforts to climb this trail can lead to sprains and fractures, just the type of memories you do not want from visiting this beautiful national park. Figure 6.21 offers some handy items that will help you stay safer when hiking. Hiking is far safer for elderly persons with an ankle or knee disability who are willing to stay away from ledges and remain on designated hiking trails (see Fig. 6.21). Terrain can be quite rough when on a hike, and planning the trip to minimize danger takes extra effort but is worthwhile. When hiking over bridges, always note the guardrails and never cross them. It is best to take an alternate path whenever balance is required.

6.4 Conclusion

Mechanical falls are often preventable by changes to the environment. This chapter has reviewed several reasons for mechanical falls. Eliminating these factors may reduce the risk of a fall in high-risk individuals. In a future chapter, we will review specific ways to reduce fall risk in vulnerable populations.

Those at risk for falling should use handrails when ascending or descending stairs, avoid slippery surfaces and use proper footwear, avoid surprise steps, uneven surfaces, wrinkled carpets, and clutter. Night-lights and grab bars are essential to prevent falls. Assistive devices such as canes, walkers, rollators, and wheelchairs should be used properly. Caregivers play a big role in the prevention of falls. The elderly should use caution, stand up slowly, and not take chances. Walking outdoors and even hiking can improve the quality of one's life, but certain precautions will make the trip safer – use walking sticks and proper footwear. Wear a hat and sunscreen. Avoid dehydration. If hiking at night, always use a headlamp. Above all, never take chances.

6.5 Outdoors

1. Use walking sticks
2. Footwear for hiking
3. The hat
4. Sunscreen
5. Stay hydrated
6. Headlamp
7. Avoid danger

References

1. Mitchell SE, Aitken SA, Court-Brown CM. The epidemiology of fractures caused by falls down stairs. ISRN Epidemiol. 2013;2013:370340. https://doi.org/10.5402/2013/370340.
2. Levine IC, Montgomery RE, Novak AC. Grab Bar use influences fall Hazard during bathtub exit. Hum Factors. 2021:187208211059860. https://doi.org/10.1177/00187208211059860.
3. Amin K, Skyving M, Bonander C, Krafft M, Nilson F. Fall- and collision-related injuries among pedestrians in road traffic environment - a Swedish national register-based study. J Saf Res. 2022;81:153–65. https://doi.org/10.1016/j.jsr.2022.02.007.
4. Oxley J, O'Hern S, Burtt D, Rossiter B. Falling while walking: a hidden contributor to pedestrian injury. Accid Anal Prev. 2018;114:77–82. https://doi.org/10.1016/j.aap.2017.01.010.
5. Rosen T, Mack KA, Noonan RK. Slipping and tripping: fall injuries in adults associated with rugs and carpets. J Inj Violence Res. 2013;5(1):61–9. https://doi.org/10.5249/jivr.v5i1.177.
6. Tarsuslu Simsek T, Tütün Yümin E, Sertel M, Öztürk A, Yümin M. Assistive device usage in elderly people and evaluation of mobility level. Topics in Geriatric Rehabilitation. 2012;28(3):190. https://doi.org/10.1097/TGR.0b013e3182581d72.
7. Mali N, Restrepo F, Abrahams A, Sands L, Goldberg DM, Gruss R, et al. Safety concerns in mobility-assistive products for older adults: content analysis of online reviews. J Med Internet Res. 2023;25:e42231. https://doi.org/10.2196/42231.
8. Bradley SM, Hernandez CR. Geriatric assistive devices. Am Fam Physician. 2011;84(4):405–11.
9. Dani M, Dirksen A, Taraborrelli P, Panagopolous D, Torocastro M, Sutton R, et al. Orthostatic hypotension in older people: considerations, diagnosis and management. Clin Med (Lond). 2021;21(3):e275–e82. https://doi.org/10.7861/clinmed.2020-1044.
10. Savvidis E, von der Decken CB. Forces acting on foot soles during stair climbing in healthy probands and in patients with coxarthrosis. Biomed Tech (Berl). 1999;44(4):98–103.
11. Rauch S, Wallner B, Ströhle M, Dal Cappello T, Brodmann MM. Climbing accidents-prospective data analysis from the international alpine trauma registry and systematic review of the literature. Int J Environ Res Public Health. 2019;17(1) https://doi.org/10.3390/ijerph17010203.
12. Sander M, Sander M, Burbidge T, Beecker J. The efficacy and safety of sunscreen use for the prevention of skin cancer. CMAJ. 2020;192(50):E1802–e8. https://doi.org/10.1503/cmaj.201085.

Chapter 7
Exercises to Prevent Falls

7.1 Introduction

Exercise is the centerpiece of this book. That is because many of the reasons people fall hinge on the well-being of their muscles, muscle memory, and bone resilience. As we age, we lose balance and muscle tone. Immobility, poor nutrition, and underlying health problems all add to the growing problem of weakness that can culminate in frailty. Although there is no warranty, the clinical evidence from prior research studies demonstrates decreased fall or injury rates in people who undergo exercise programs. It also helps improve the quality of life, self-confidence, and independence.

This chapter will highlight features adapted from two well-established programs, the Otago Exercise Program (OEP) and Fitness and Mobility Exercise (FAME) Program.

OEP has been tested in frail persons and FAME from those recovering from strokes. They can be modified for each person's needs. When initiating an exercise program, persons with a significant disability should first meet with a rehabilitation team that includes a physical therapist. Afterward, one might wish to use a personal trainer who has been certified in senior fitness to continue the program on an ongoing basis.

In addition, this chapter will highlight several exercises that can be incorporated with OEP and FAME. These are divided into stretching, lower body strength, balance, and core strength improvement. Finally, this chapter will introduce you to some fun community projects that help maintain fitness – senior soccer and pickleball.

In the appendix, you will find a more in-depth discussion of how muscles work and why we want to condition them (also if aging leads to falls, what causes aging?).

7.2 Otago Exercise Program (OEP)

This is a home-based fall prevention program that incorporates balance and strength exercises to prevent falls. It is designed to be administered by a licensed physical therapist and can be tailored to individual patients. It was initially designed for people over 80 years old with a history of falls and works best for frail adults. It is also useful for deconditioned adults and persons with chronic diseases. The CDC and the National Center for Injury Prevention and Control (NCIPC) have adopted the program that was initially developed in New Zealand.

The program consists of 5 strengthening (Fig. 7.1) and 12 balance exercises (Figs. 7.2 and 7.3), starting at 10 repetitions. They are to be performed three times a week. As one progresses, the number of repetitions can be increased, and ankle weights can be used. Walking for around 1 h a week in two 30-min sessions or smaller and more frequent 10-min sessions is part of the program.

The program has been validated in four trials. It reduced falls by 30% to 66% and reduced fall-related injuries by 28%. About 70% of participants continued the program after the year study period ended [1].

7.2 Otago Exercise Program (OEP)

1-Front knee strengthening	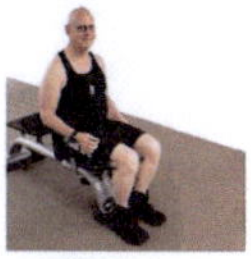 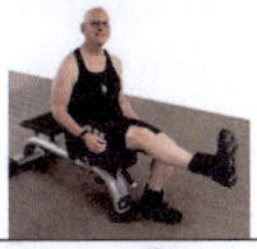	This can be done with ankle weights. • Sit in a chair. • Straighten the leg as much as possible, then lower the leg. • Repeat ten times. • Repeat with the other leg.
2-Back knee strengthening	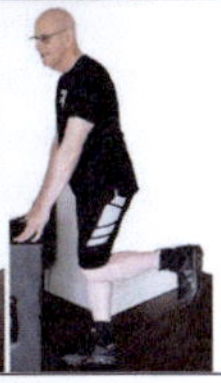 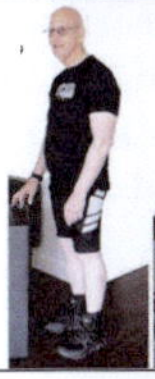	This exercise can be done with ankle weights. • Stand up facing a table. • Bend the knee and bring up your foot to your buttocks. • Return to standing. • Repeat ten times and then perform with the other knee.
3-Side hip strengthening	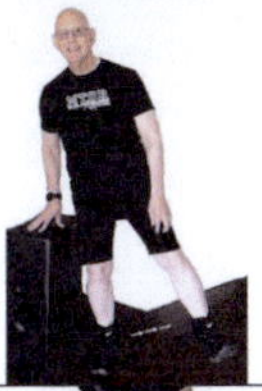	This exercise can be done with ankle weights. • Stand up with a hand on a table. • Lift one leg out to the side and return. • Repeat 10 times. • Turn around and repeat 10 times with the other leg. • This exercise can be done with elastics also (see below).
4-Calf raise	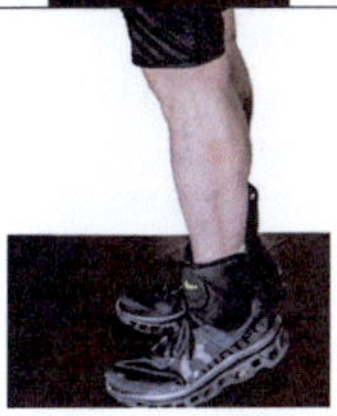	Calf raises can be done with and without support. • Stand up and face the table. (With support your hand should rest on the table). Tuck in your core • Keep your feet at shoulder-width. • Lift your heels, standing on your toes. • Then return your heels to the ground. • Repeat 10 times.
5-Toe raises	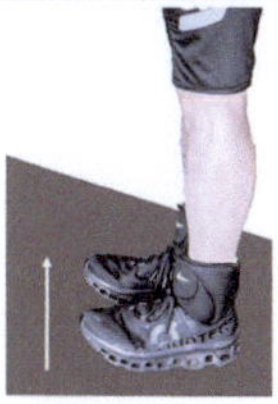	Toe raises can be done with and without support. • Stand up and face the table. (When support is needed your hand should rest on the table). Tuck in your core. • Keep your feet at shoulder-width. • Come back on your heels raising your toes. • Lower your toes. • Repeat 10 times.

Fig. 7.1 Otago Strength Exercises

1-Knee bends	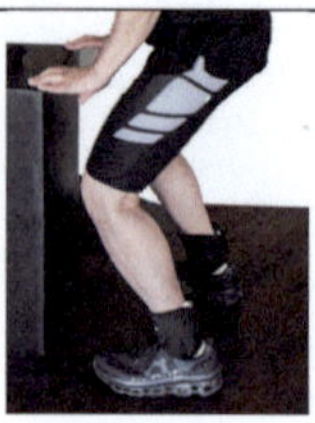	This can be done with and without support. • Stand up, face the table, and tuck in your core. • If support is needed, keep both hands on the table. • The feet should be shoulder-width apart. • Squat down half way, bending your knees. • Your knees extend over the toes. • Straighten up when your heels start to lift. • Repeat 10 times.
2-Backwards walking	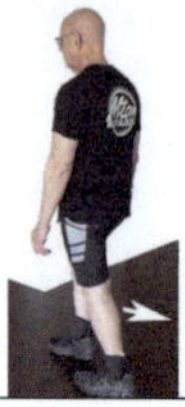	This can be done with or without support • Stand up tall and tuck in your core. • Walk backwards 10 steps. • Turn around and repeat.
3-Walking and turning around	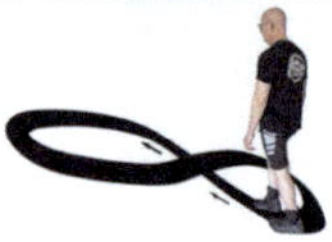	• While walking at a regular pace with your core tucked in, turn clockwise, and walk back to the starting position making a figure of 8. • Repeat walking counter-clockwise.
4-Sideways walking	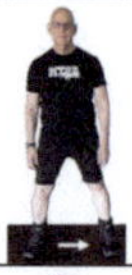	• While standing tall with your core tucked in and your hands on or by your hips take 10 side steps. • Now take 10 side steps in the opposite direction.
5-Heel to toe stand	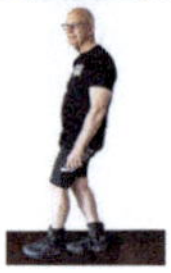	This can be done with or without support. • Place one foot in front of the other in a straight line. • The heel of one foot should touch the toes of the other. • Hold this position for 10 seconds and then change feet and repeat

Fig. 7.2 Otago Balance Exercises (Part 1)

7.2 Otago Exercise Program (OEP)

Exercise	Description
6-Heel to toe walk	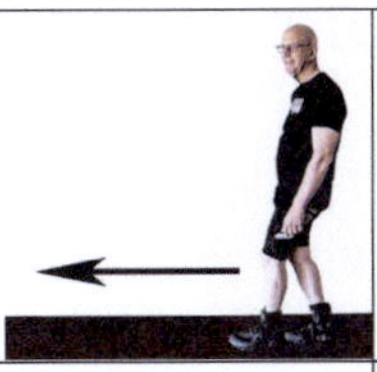 This can be done with or without support. • Stand up with the core tight. • Place one foot in front of the other in a straight line. • Take 10 steps. • Turn around and repeat
7-Stand on one leg	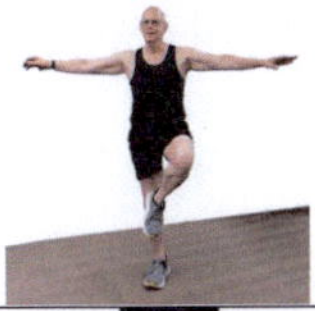 This can be done with or without support. • While standing on one leg try to hold this position for 10-30 seconds. • Repeat with the other leg.
8-Heel walking	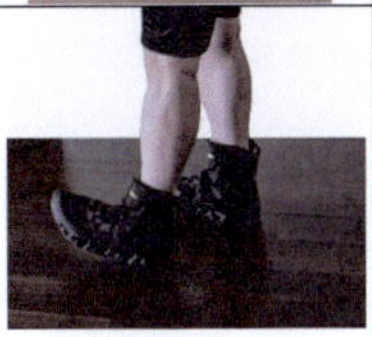 This can be done with and without support. • Stand up tall beside a table. • Hold on to the table if support is needed. • Step forward coming back on the heel. • After ten steps lower feet to the ground and turn around. • Repeat.
9-Toe Walking	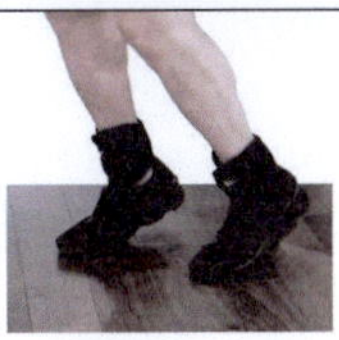 This can be done with and without support. • Stand up tall beside a table. • Hold on to the table if support is needed. • Place one heel in front of the other toe and take 10 steps. • Lower the heels and turn around. • Repeat.
10-Heel Toe Walking backwards	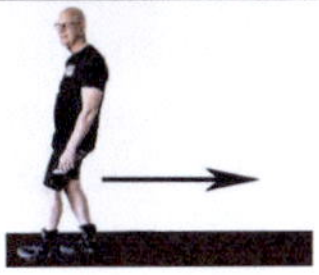 Make sure you are near a table or wall for support. Make certain there is a clear path behind you. • Stand up tall and place the toe directly behind the heel. • Repeat for 10 steps. • Turn around and repeat.
11-Sit to stand	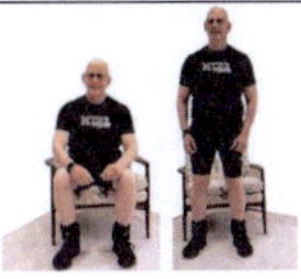 This can be done with two hands, one hand, or no hands. • Sit on a chair. • Place your feet behind the knees. • Lean forward. • Move to a standing position, and then sit back down. • The number of times to repeat this varies from individual to individual.
12-Stair walking (using siderails)	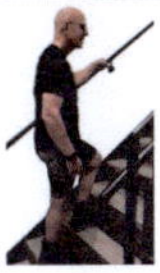 Hold handrail at all times. • Walk up and back down a set of stairs. • The number of stairs varies .from individual to individual • Walking up the stairs can build up the muscles in the back of the leg and the gluteus area while walking down the stairs can help rebuild and strengthen bone.

Fig. 7.3 Otago Balance Exercises (Part 2)

7.3 Fitness and Mobility Exercise (FAME)

The Fitness and Mobility Exercise (FAME) Program for stroke has been developed and validated as being beneficial in improving complications caused by strokes in the elderly [2]. Selective muscle strengthening exercises have improved post-strength muscle strength in some patients. This program uses weights and elastic bands. The program considers that stroke patients often fall onto the side that is the weakest and that because of immobility, bones are fragile. Also, patients who require assistance when standing will need a caregiver who has been trained in assisting stroke patients to assist with the exercises. The program is designed for physical therapists and occupational therapists and is made up of four parts (see Figs. 7.4, 7.5, 7.6, and 7.7). It is a 1-hour group program repeated two to three times weekly for at least 4 months. Self-directed home exercises, especially walking, should accompany the program. Patients should be screened by their physician and, if necessary, have a stress test to determine any cardiac limitations. The program starts with a 10-min warm-up period followed by stretching exercises. It then focuses on strength, balance, agility, and aerobic fitness. Most strength training exercises are done standing to force weight-bearing. Balance and agility include tai-chi-like movements. Here are some illustrated examples of the FAME program. The exercises start with 2 sets, 5 repetitions each, and progress to 2 sets of 10 repetitions.

The maximum target heart rate (MTHR) varies by age and historically was 220 minus the age in years. The newer MTHR is calculated by subtracting the age times 0.7 from 207. Thus, a 75-year-old person would have a maximum heart rate around 155. If the resting heart rate for this individual is 75, then the heart rate reserve (HRR), the difference between the MTHR and the resting heart rate, is 80. The program starts with a 40%–50% of HRR and progresses to 70%–80% of HRR Thus, our 75-year-old would start with a target of $75 + 32 = 107$ to $75 + 64 = 139$ beats per minute. Participants should be screened with a treadmill test by a cardiologist, and this regimen first discussed with the doctor. The FAME program has been validated to improve stroke balance and muscle function, cardiovascular fitness, and bone density [3].

Many of the exercises are the same as in the Otago Exercise Program. The program also emphasizes socialization.

7.3 Fitness and Mobility Exercise (FAME)

1-Sit to stand	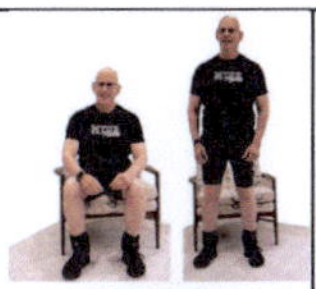	This can be done with two hands, one hand or no hands. • Sit on a chair. • Place feet behind the knees. • Lean forward. • Move to a standing position, and then sit back down. • Repeat.
2-Standing, rise on toes	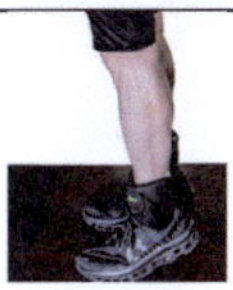	Calf raises – can be done with and without support. • Stand up and face the table. (Rest your hands on the table for support). • Tuck in your core. • Keep your feet at shoulder-width. • Lift your heels, standing on your toes. • Then return your heels to the ground. • Repeat.
3-Standing, lift toes and rise on heels	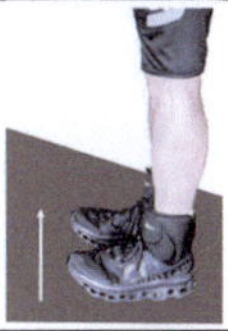	Toe raises – can be done with and without support. • Stand up and face the table. (With support, your hand should rest on the table). Tuck in your core. • Keep your feet at shoulder-width. • Come back on your heels raising your toes. • Lower your toes. • Repeat.
4-Standing push up against the wall	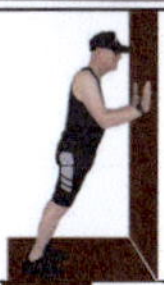	• Lean forward, keeping the body straight. • Lower body into the wall until your chest nearly touches. • Push back to the original position. • Repeat.
5-Standing, back against the wall, bend knees and hold	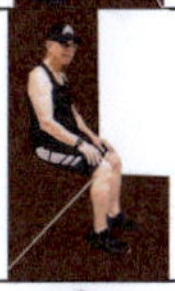	• Start with your back against the wall. • Your fees should be around 2 feet from the wall. • The knees should be over your ankles. • Sit against the wall for 20 to 60 seconds. • Slide back up the wall.
6-Fast walking	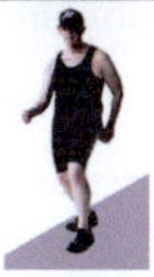	• Stand tall with head up and chin parallel to the ground. • Hold shoulders down and back. • Walk briskly swinging your arms. • Engage your core. Step from heel to toe. • Try to increase your pace gradually. • Goal is to walk 100 steps per minute for 30 minutes. • Wear a hat.
7-Walk with long steps	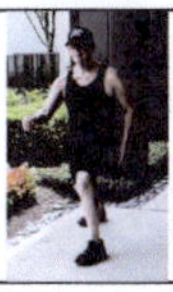	• Stand tall, engage your core, keep your chin up, shoulders down and back. • Walk briskly taking giant strides.

Fig. 7.4 Strength (FAME Part 1)

1-Fast walking	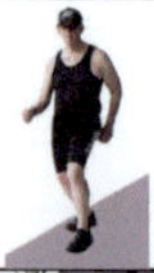	See above.
2-Walking with long steps	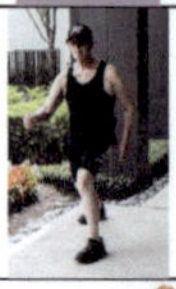	See above.
3-Sit to stand	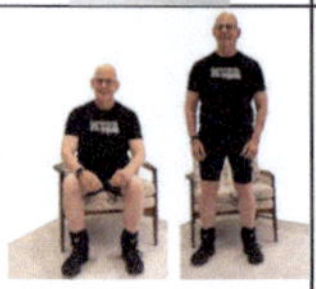	This can be done with two hands, one hand or no hands. • Sit on a chair. • Place feet behind the knees. • Lean forward. • Move to a standing position, and then sit back down. • Some people will take longer. • Repeat.

Fig. 7.5 Endurance and Fitness (FAME Part 2)

1-Step up on the stepper, then back down (two feet)	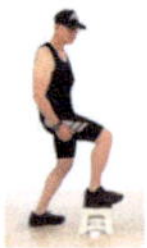	• Step onto the step with both feet. • Then step back down on the other side. • Then step back down and repeat.
2-Step sideways on the stepper (2 feet) then step back down on the other side	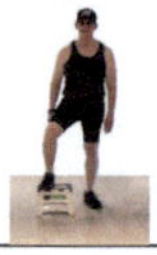	• Step sideways onto the step. • Now step up with the other foot. • Then step back down **on the opposite side, and repeat.**
3-Stand and do a quick lunge on command (Stationary lunge)	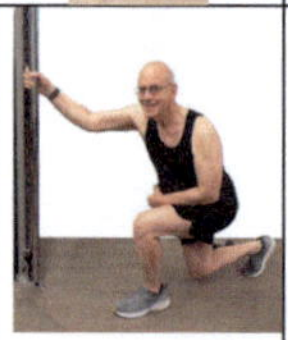	• From a forward position drop the body straight down. • The knee stays behind the toes. Keep the weight on the heel. • Bend your knees to what your range of motion allows. • Engage your core and exhale while coming back to the starting position. • Straighten your legs when coming up, but keep them staggered for balance. • Repeat.
4-Try to push the instructor off balance	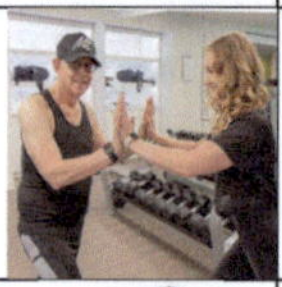	• Balance your hands against the instructor's. • Push hard and try to throw her off balance.
5-Rise from the chair, walk around the chair, then sit back down.	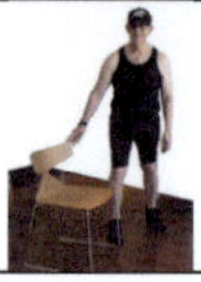	• Stand up from the chair then walk around it clockwise. • Next, walk from the chair counter clockwise.

Fig. 7.6 Agility (FAME Part 3)

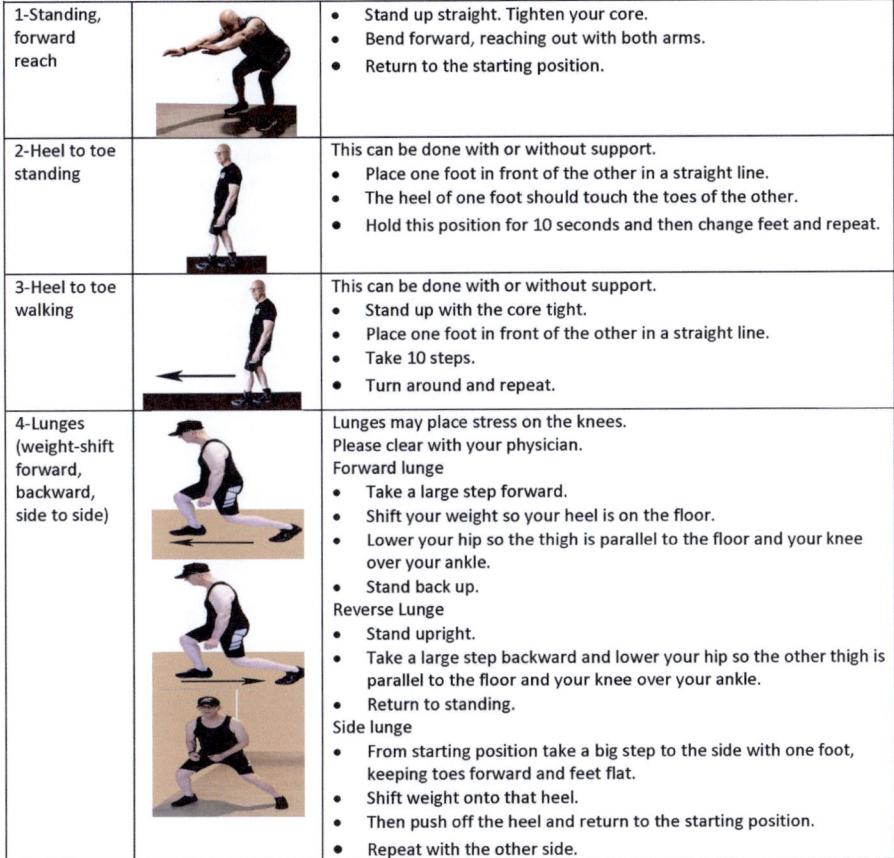

1-Standing, forward reach		• Stand up straight. Tighten your core. • Bend forward, reaching out with both arms. • Return to the starting position.
2-Heel to toe standing		This can be done with or without support. • Place one foot in front of the other in a straight line. • The heel of one foot should touch the toes of the other. • Hold this position for 10 seconds and then change feet and repeat.
3-Heel to toe walking		This can be done with or without support. • Stand up with the core tight. • Place one foot in front of the other in a straight line. • Take 10 steps. • Turn around and repeat.
4-Lunges (weight-shift forward, backward, side to side)		Lunges may place stress on the knees. Please clear with your physician. Forward lunge • Take a large step forward. • Shift your weight so your heel is on the floor. • Lower your hip so the thigh is parallel to the floor and your knee over your ankle. • Stand back up. Reverse Lunge • Stand upright. • Take a large step backward and lower your hip so the other thigh is parallel to the floor and your knee over your ankle. • Return to standing. Side lunge • From starting position take a big step to the side with one foot, keeping toes forward and feet flat. • Shift weight onto that heel. • Then push off the heel and return to the starting position. • Repeat with the other side.

Fig. 7.7 Balance Exercises (FAME Part 4)

7.4 Additional Exercises

Robust and healthy persons who are not at direct risk for falling should also exercise regularly to maintain and improve balance and muscle strength. Exercises can be performed during the day and squeezed into free time. This is known as a fitness snack. Aging can be associated with muscle loss, but this can be reduced with resistance exercises. Exercises can be designed to strengthen the central or core muscles and those of the lower extremities. By practicing balance through exercise, one can help restore the muscle memory that is associated with equilibrium. Several practical exercises presented in *Staying Healthy with Kidney Disease* are highlighted here. This exercise program was developed by Senior Fitness Specialist Michelle L. (Misha) Nguyen to help augment balance and preserve muscle [4, 5]. Personal trainers Kane Bryant and Alyssa Conway also lent their expertise to this project. Several clinical trials have demonstrated that exercise is a valuable way to reduce falls [6]. The additional exercises is divided into five parts, starting with stretching (see Fig. 7.8).

1-Quad stretch		• Stand up tall, engage the core, and hold a sturdy surface for balance. • Grab one foot and pull towards your rear, keeping thighs and knees together. • This stretch can also be performed lying on your side, hips aligned so one is above the other, pulling the leg that is on top. • Try to hold the stretch for 20 sec before switching legs.
2-Pyriform stretch		• While lying on your back, Lift your left leg and cross it over just above the right knee. • Grab your left ankle with your right hand. • Now grab your right ankle with your left hand. • Pull both ankles. • This stretch can be performed at least once per day up to three times per day.
3-Split hamstring stretch		• Sit on the floor with your legs apart in front of you, and feet against the wall. • Keep your legs as straight as possible. • Reach for the wall. • Keep your body straight and tall. • Do not over-stretch for risk of muscle, tendon, or ligament damage. • Hold stretch position for at least 15 seconds. • Repeat as desired. • Great way to end a session!
4-Child's pose		• Spread your knees and let your belly fall to your thighs. • Relax all parts of your body. • Move your forehead to the floor and extend out your hands, palms down, as far as you can. • Breathe deeply. • This is best done on an empty stomach.
5-Cat cow stretch		• (Meow) Exhale and round your spine upward, keeping your belly tucked toward the spine, dropping your head and chin. Look toward your belly. • Drive your belly toward your spine. • (Moo) Inhale deeply and arch your back down as much as you can while moving your head upward.
6-Shoulder stretch		• This exercise is for shoulder pain. If you do not have an exercise ball, use a chair. • Reach forward. • The arm should not be higher than the shoulder. • Push your arm into the ball and hold for 10 to 30 seconds.
7-Knee and calve stretch		• When your hands against the wall and your toe near the wall extend, driving the knee forward with your knee. • The heel should stay on the ground.

Fig. 7.8 Additional exercises: Stretching

7.4.1 Core (See Fig. 7.9)

The core is a group of central muscles in the body and is made up of abdominal muscles, muscles of the hip, spine, and back. It stabilizes the body and improves balance and posture, allowing the body to rotate and maintain momentum. A strong core can help prevent fall injuries and decrease back pain.

7.4 Additional Exercises

1-Planks	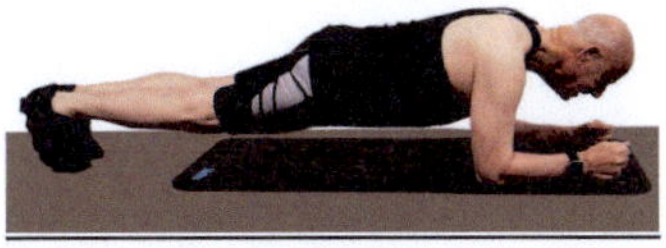	• Start face down. Do not hunch or drop head. Do not bend legs. • Hollow the chest and spread shoulder blades wide. • Only forearms and toes should touch the floor. • Beginners can start on their knees. • Aim for a nearly horizontal position and do not let your body drop too low or raise too high. • Push your shoulder blades toward the ground. • Tuck in the tail bone, keep the core sight. • Tilt your pelvis back and squeeze your glutes to engage the core. • Try to hold for 15 seconds, and extend to 60 seconds once your form is correct. Keep your form. Breathe deeply. • Do not get up too soon!
2-Bicycle crunch	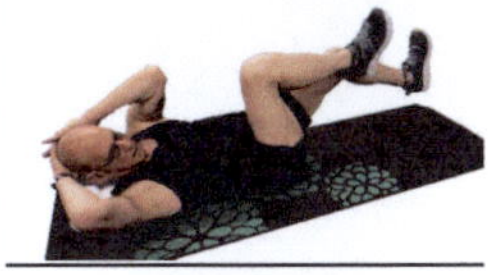	• Keep your shoulders off the floor and contract your core muscles. • Pull back a shoulder blade and raise the knees 90 degrees off the floor. • Rotate the torso with opposite extensions. • Try to touch your elbow to the opposite knee by twisting upward. • Alternate twisting and pumping.
3-Reverse crunch	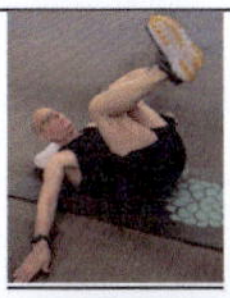	• Lie down on back with knees bent • Arms to the side or behind your head for support. • Exhale while bringing knees toward the chest and • Raise the hips off the floor. • Hold in a reverse crunched position • Inhale as you return to starting position. Repeat. Start with 3 sets of 8–10 reps and increase reps as you improve
4-Bird dog	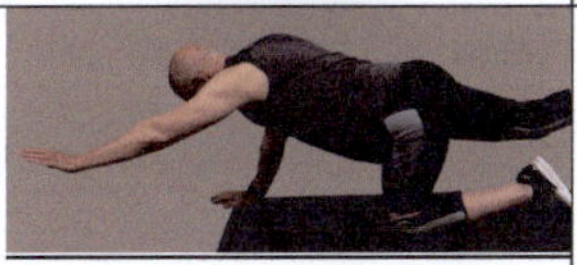	• Start on your hands and knees (table pose) • Focus on forming a straight line from your hand down to your toes. Do not let your chest sag or your back curve excessively. • Extend one hand and the opposite leg, Keep hips square thighs square to the mat. • Return to the table pose and repeat on the other side for 10 reps on each side
5-Scissors	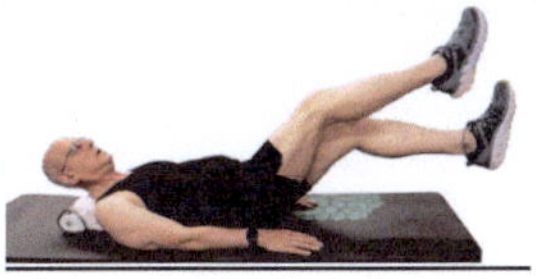	• Lie on your back with your hands at your side . • You can place them underneath your glutes for back support. • Engage your core and press your lower back against the mat. • Only lower legs as far as able to keep lower back pressed into the mat. A lift or arch in the back means you went too far. • Extend your legs straight out, and twist them above each other or straight up and down. • Advance to 3 sets of 45 seconds.

Fig. 7.9 Additional exercises: Core

7.4.2 Lower Body Strength (See Fig. 7.10)

Lower body exercises are critical to preserve health. Strong thigh muscles can protect the knee joints and help catch and maintain balance. The sit to stand and stationary supported lunge were mentioned above.

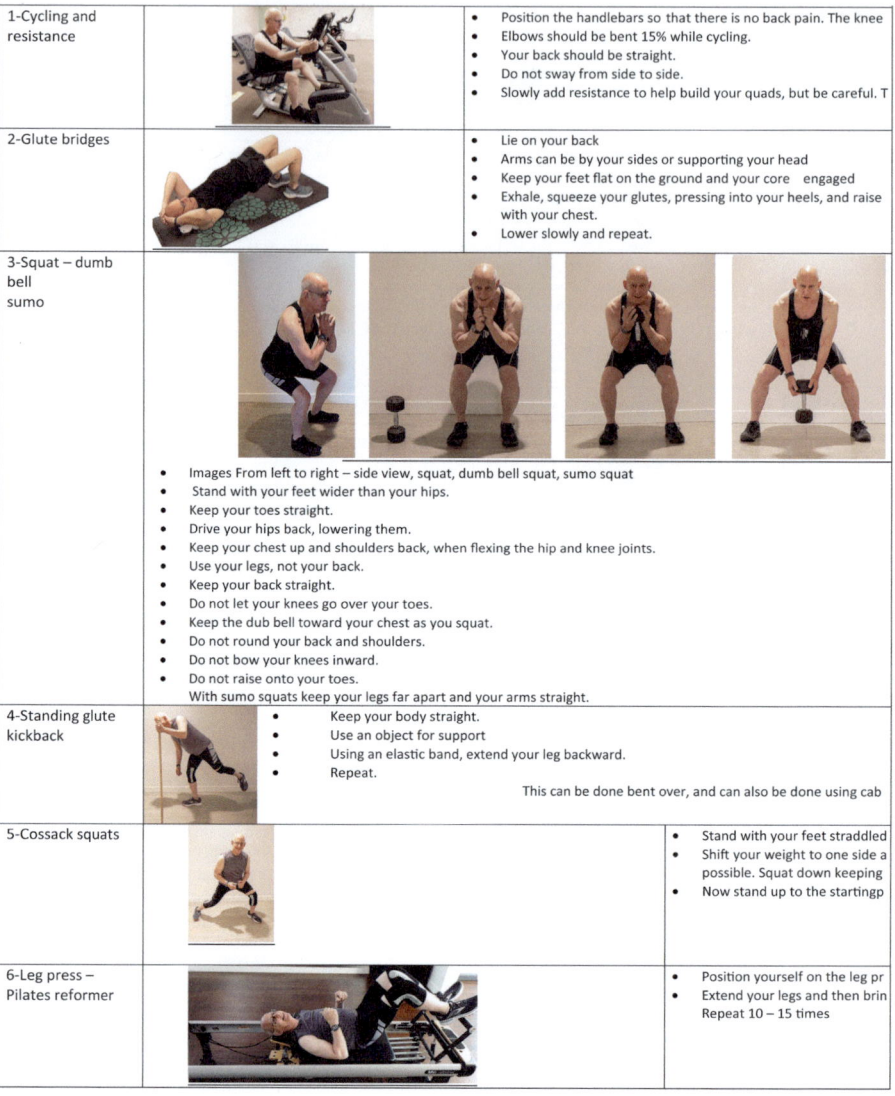

Fig. 7.10 Additional exercises: Lower body strength

7.4 Additional Exercises

7.4.3 Balance (See Fig. 7.11)

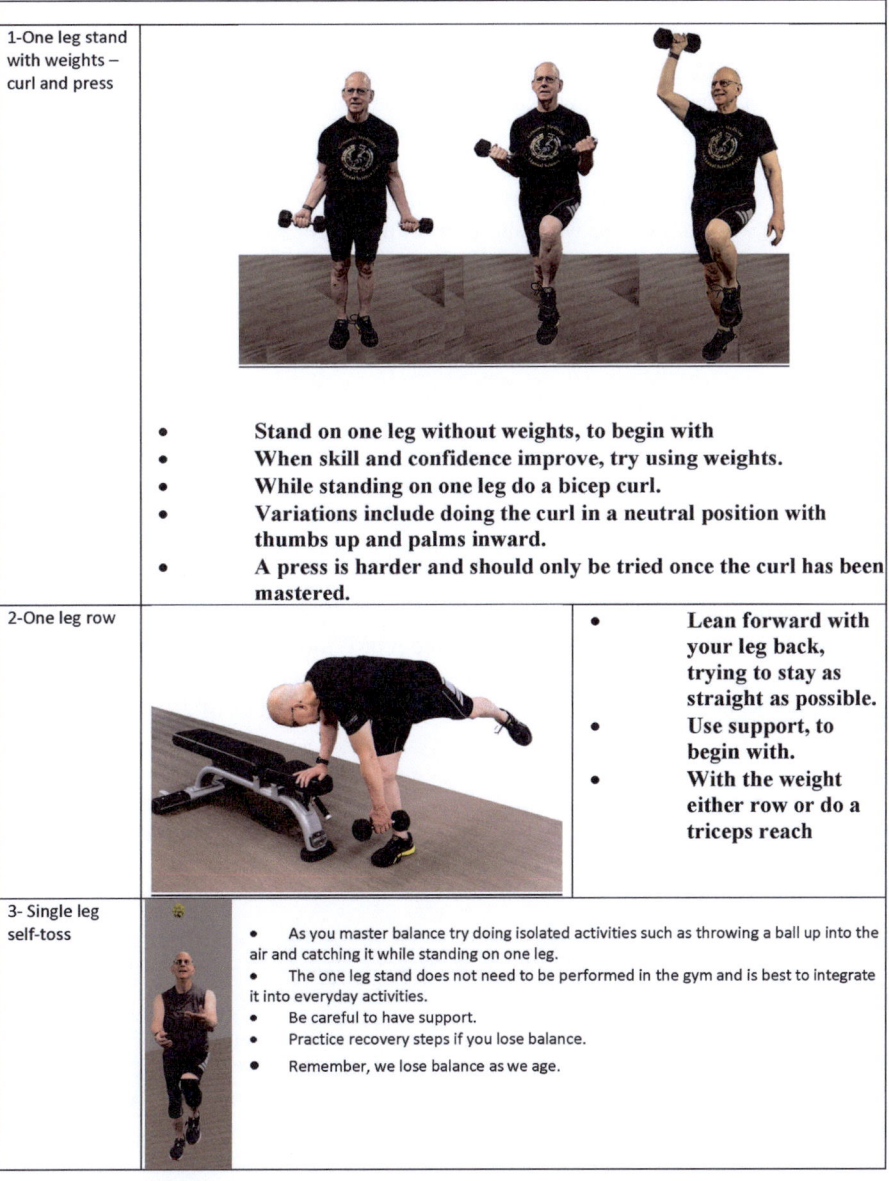

Fig. 7.11 Additional exercises: Balance

7.4.4 Recovery Step Exercises (See Fig. 7.12)

- Lean forward until you feel off-balance.
- Step forward with one foot in front of you until you have reestablished balance. Repeat this ten times. Perform the same exercise with the other foot. Next, try stepping backward ten times, first with the left and then the right foot.
- Next, when feeling off-balance, step across with one foot until you have reestablished balance.
- Finally, stand with your feet together, then lean to the side until you feel off-balance. Step to the side with one foot until you regain balance. When you feel comfortable, you can practice "falling" and regaining balance without holding onto anything.

7.5 Fitness Snacks

Many people fail to meet CDC guideline recommendations for daily physical activity; they are too busy (**https://www.cdc.gov/physicalactivity/index.html**)! Lack of time is the most frequent obstacle to getting enough exercise [7]. An exercise snack is defined as ≤1 min of intense exercise that is performed periodically during the day. These are well tolerated and may help promote fitness in these busy individuals who otherwise would remain inactive at sedentary jobs [8]. Fitness snacks are all-out but brief exercises. Just one "snack" daily will probably be useless; more are needed [9]. Recommendations support either extended snacks of 2 10-min bouts per day or 3 to 8 60-s bouts of vigorous exercise [10].

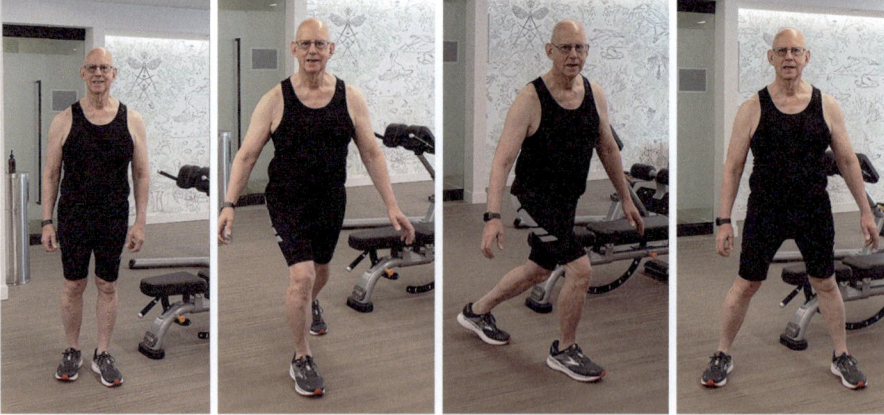

Fig. 7.12 How to land to prevent serious injury when falling. Several recovery steps taken unexpectedly getting off-balance may help offset the gravitational force of a fall. These maneuvers may not always prevent a fall but may be helpful

7.6 Soccer and Pickleball (See Fig. 7.13)

Inactivity is a major problem in persons over 75 years old. It is estimated that 49% of people this age and older are inactive (**https://www.independentliving.co.uk/advice/adapted-sports-older-people/**). Adapting sports for older people has many advantages and is used to improve socialization and fitness. In the United Kingdom, where soccer is the national sport as opposed to American football, a modified game called walking football has been around since 1932. It differs from customary soccer in that games last 60 instead of 90 mins, unlimited substitutions are allowed, and there are 7 players instead of 11. No running or contact is allowed. Several other sports, including volleyball, have also been adapted.

In prediabetic persons aged 55–70 years, a 16-week program of exercise, and dietary change, including participation in senior soccer teams, were compared to dietary change alone. Although the blood sugar measurements improved in both groups, the VO_2 max (the maximum amount of oxygen delivered to muscles during full-throttle exercise, considered the best indicator of cardiovascular fitness) increased 14% when exercise sports were added. Blood pressure and fat stores declined significantly with exercise [11].

Pickleball is an emerging sport that is attracting attention, especially among older adults. It is popular where seniors congregate or live, from country clubs to retirement centers. It is played on a 20 × 44 ft. hard court with a paddle and a special ball and combines many of the attributes of badminton, ping pong, and tennis. The game involves moderate to vigorous play and helps meet exercise guidelines. It can positively impact participants' fitness, well-being, and psychological well-being [12–15]. Yet, its popularity may hide that significant injuries such as sprains, strains, and fractures can occur. Tendon tears are debilitating but can and do occur during vigorous play. Serious eye injuries have been reported, and eye protection is necessary [16]. Some injuries can be prevented with a better sense of awareness. Many injuries are from overuse and involve the shoulder, knee, ankle, back elbow, and back. Serious hamstring tears have been reported. While shoulder, foot, and wrist

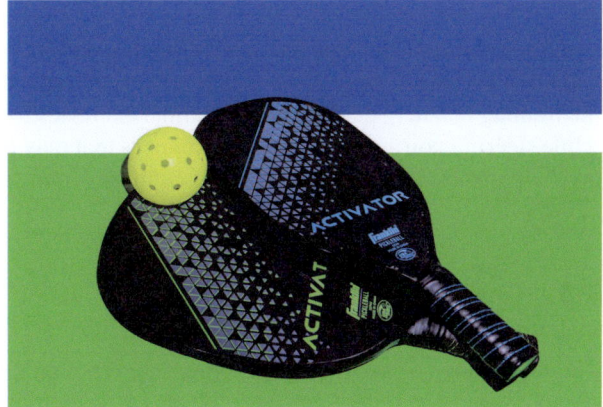

Fig. 7.13 Pickleball is a popular sport for seniors but can lead to injury if not properly prepared or coached

injuries are most common in women, men tend to have injuries to the knees, ankles, thighs, and calves. Warm-up recommendations have been published and include a range of motion and quadriceps stretches (**https://www.paddletek.com/blogs/news/5-pickleball-warmups**). Adequate hydration is also necessary. There are lessons and skills that can be acquired with coaching and training that can improve form, enhance performance, and reduce the risk of injury. Athletic positions are common for most sports and ensure proper stability and footing. Training includes avoiding sudden stops and overcompensation. Since older persons have less ability to turn, they try to backpedal on their heels to return a lob shot going over their head. Impaired balance and proprioception can result in an injurious fall. Part of pickleball coaching should involve learning to fall and roll with the momentum rather than extending the hand, leading to a fractured wrist. Since pickleball service is underhanded, damage to rotator cuffs can be minimized. Coaching should also include how to choose and grip the paddle. Players should use shoes designed for the hard court action of pickleball instead of running shoes. These sneakers must handle quick movements in any direction, and thus, the outsoles need to be strong and the tread pattern responsive. Lateral stability helps prevent injuries to the ankles and knees. These shoes should have a wide base and stiff lower structure to ensure stability [17–19]. When exercising, the goal is to improve mobility and endurance, muscle strength, balance, and independence. Cutting corners with equipment, training, or warming up can lead to less optimal outcomes.

7.7 Using a Trainer

Exercises must be done correctly to do what they are intended to while avoiding injurious sprains or strains. Having incorrect form or misjudging which weight to use can lead to injury, especially in the elderly, where range of motion may be compromised. Since we cannot see ourselves exercising, it is best to have an experienced person on hand who can coach and give us feedback. The physical therapist is essential for recovering from a medical condition, but after the formal physical therapy session has ended, one may benefit from continued exercise. A personal trainer can identify the muscle groups that need targeting and help you set up a more effective and safer exercise program. Also, given that osteoarthritis is common in the elderly, the training can help determine the optimal exercises that will help protect the joints while steering you away from those exercises that may produce harm. A good trainer can help inspire intrinsic motivation, confidence, and self-satisfaction.

7.8 Conclusion

The importance of exercise to a program designed to reduce falling cannot be overstated. Exercising in persons with fall risk will help improve muscle strength, balance, and coordination. To be effective, exercise programs should be well thought out and planned. The Otago Exercise Program and the Fitness and Mobility Exercise Program have been validated to help improve fall risks in persons who are frail or who have had a stroke. More robust persons might wish to try additional exercises, some of which are outlined in this chapter. Sometimes people are too busy to designate a specific period of time to train. A few brief exercise periods of 1 min each may suffice. Group activities such as pickleball may also improve fitness, lessening the chance of falling. Training alongside a highly experienced person can give you added insight, help avoid injuries, and improve motivation.

References

1. Robertson MC, Campbell AJ, Gardner MM, Devlin N. Preventing injuries in older people by preventing falls: a meta-analysis of individual-level data. J Am Geriatr Soc. 2002;50(5):905–11. https://doi.org/10.1046/j.1532-5415.2002.50218.x.
2. Pang MY, Eng JJ, Dawson AS, McKay HA, Harris JE. A community-based fitness and mobility exercise program for older adults with chronic stroke: a randomized, controlled trial. J Am Geriatr Soc. 2005;53(10):1667–74. https://doi.org/10.1111/j.1532-5415.2005.53521.x.
3. Eng JJ. Fitness and mobility exercise (FAME) program for stroke. Top Geriatr Rehabil. 2010;26(4):310–23. https://doi.org/10.1097/TGR.0b013e3181fee736.
4. Nguyen ML, Fadem SZ. Exercises for people with chronic kidney disease and seniors. In: Fadem SZ, editor. Staying healthy with kidney disease: a complete guide for patients. Cham: Springer International Publishing; 2022. p. 87–101.
5. Fadem SZ. Falls in CKD patients and seniors: causes and prevention. In: Fadem SZ, editor. Staying healthy with kidney disease: a complete guide for patients. Cham: Springer International Publishing; 2022. p. 103–12.
6. Sherrington C, Michaleff ZA, Fairhall N, Paul SS, Tiedemann A, Whitney J, et al. Exercise to prevent falls in older adults: an updated systematic review and meta-analysis. Br J Sports Med. 2017;51(24):1750. https://doi.org/10.1136/bjsports-2016-096547.
7. Hoare E, Stavreski B, Jennings GL, Kingwell BA. Exploring motivation and barriers to physical activity among active and inactive Australian adults. Sports (Basel). 2017;5(3) https://doi.org/10.3390/sports5030047.
8. Islam H, Gibala MJ, Little JP. Exercise snacks: a novel strategy to improve Cardiometabolic health. Exerc Sport Sci Rev. 2022;50(1):31–7. https://doi.org/10.1249/jes.0000000000000275.
9. Songsorn P, Lambeth-Mansell A, Mair JL, Haggett M, Fitzpatrick BL, Ruffino J, et al. Exercise training comprising of single 20-s cycle sprints does not provide a sufficient stimulus for improving maximal aerobic capacity in sedentary individuals. Eur J Appl Physiol. 2016;116(8):1511–7. https://doi.org/10.1007/s00421-016-3409-8.
10. Huang CH, Yen M. Applying an exercise snack-based health promotion strategy. Hu Li Za Zhi. 2023;70(2):78–83. https://doi.org/10.6224/jn.202304_70(2).10.
11. Katsuyama M, Higo E, Miyamoto M, Nakamae T, Onitsuka D, Fukumoto A, et al. Development of prevention strategies against bath-related deaths based on epidemiological surveys of inquest records in Kagoshima prefecture. Sci Rep. 2023;13(1):2277. https://doi.org/10.1038/s41598-023-29400-7.
12. Webber SC, Anderson S, Biccum L, Jin S, Khawashki S, Tittlemier BJ. Physical activity intensity of singles and doubles Pickleball in older adults. J Aging Phys Act 2022:1–6. doi: https://doi.org/10.1123/japa.2022-0194, 31, 365.
13. Cerezuela JL, Lirola MJ, Cangas AJ. Pickleball and mental health in adults: a systematic review. Front Psychol. 2023;14:1137047. https://doi.org/10.3389/fpsyg.2023.1137047.
14. Ryu J, Heo J, Lee S. Pickleball, personality, and Eudaimonic Well-being in middle-aged and older adults. J Aging Phys Act. 2022;30(5):885–92. https://doi.org/10.1123/japa.2021-0298.

15. Wray P, Ward CK, Nelson C, Sulzer SH, Dakin CJ, Thompson BJ, et al. Pickleball for inactive mid-life and older adults in rural Utah: a feasibility study. Int J Environ Res Public Health. 2021;18(16) https://doi.org/10.3390/ijerph18168374.
16. Huang H, Greven MA. Traumatic lens subluxation from Pickleball injury: a case series. Retin Cases Brief Rep. 2022;Publish Ahead of Print https://doi.org/10.1097/icb.0000000000001312.
17. Weiss H, Dougherty J, DiMaggio C. Non-fatal senior pickleball and tennis-related injuries treated in United States emergency departments, 2010-2019. Inj Epidemiol. 2021;8(1):34. https://doi.org/10.1186/s40621-021-00327-9.
18. Changstrom B, McBride A, Khodaee M. Epidemiology of racket and paddle sports-related injuries treated in the United States emergency departments, 2007-2016. Phys Sportsmed. 2022;50(3):197–204. https://doi.org/10.1080/00913847.2021.1892467.
19. Vitale K, Liu S. Pickleball: review and clinical recommendations for this fast-growing sport. Curr Sports Med Rep. 2020;19(10):406–13. https://doi.org/10.1249/jsr.0000000000000759.

Chapter 8
Tai-Chi Chuan and Fall Prevention

8.1 Introduction

Falls are now the leading cause of death among those who visit the emergency room. In a cohort of 21,340 patients, the average age was 78.6 years old. About 50.2% of patients had more than one visit; 36% died within a year [1]. Throughout this book, we have emphasized that exercise reduces the risk of falls. Traditional Tai Chi programs, based on ancient martial arts, combine fitness with mindfulness, allowing participants to learn relaxing and calming techniques while improving their exercise capacity. Tai Chi Chuan, or traditional Tai Chi, includes a set of strength and balance-training exercises that are especially effective at preventing falls [2, 3]. They focus on strength, balance, breathing, flexibility, and mobility. Peter Wayne, faculty editor of the Harvard Special Health Report and the director of the Osher Center for Integrative Medicine at Brigham and Women's Hospital, has developed a special fascination with Tai Chi, collaborating to author the Harvard Medical School Guide to Tai Chi. This guide is a valuable resource to those who, after reading this chapter, are inspired to consider Tai Chi [4].

8.2 Supporting Research

8.2.1 Individual Vs Traditional Tai Chi

We often hear about the different types of Tai Chi, and this can be a source of confusion. Breaking away from traditional Tai Chi is a newer type designed for individual adaptation. Individualized Tai Chi (iTC) takes a more personalized approach than Tai Chi Chuan (tTC), tailoring the needs to meet the needs of individuals. This customization is particularly effective in an elderly population with specific health and range of motion limitations. A clinical trial randomized participants to either iTC or tTC reported that the Berg Balance Scale (BBS), a functional balance test, and muscle strength of hips and ankles were improved in the traditional Tai Chi (tTC). In contrast, in all functional balance tests, specifically the BBS, the timed up-and-go (TUG) test discussed in a previous chapter, the functional reach test, and measurements of lower-extremity strength improved significantly in the iTC group. The authors concluded by reporting that the prescription for Tai Chi should be personalized to the individual needs of the patient with respect to both intensity and difficulty [1].

8.2.2 Social Isolation

As persons age, social isolation and depression also contribute to poor outcomes. Tai Chi is an effective method to reduce falls when used as a single intervention, and it is effective in home-based training. But it may also have a role in improving the impact of social isolation on some of the adverse outcomes associated with aging. It is projected that by 2030, 20% of the US population will be over 65 years old, often struggling with chronic health conditions. Loneliness and social isolation are multifactorial challenges that face the elderly in addition to these chronic conditions. It is a promising nonpharmacologic intervention. All five styles available in modern practice integrate a balanced, holistic life path with mindfulness. It is considered a spiritual exercise program that also benefits mental health. It is being started in church groups and may emerge as a popular group activity in community centers [5, 6].

A large review of the published medical literature identified participants over 70 years of age. Tai Chi was shown to have benefits in impacting strength, flexibility, cardiovascular endurance, body composition, activities of daily living, self-esteem, and quality of life. It also impacted depression and the fear of falling [7].

8.2.3 Postural Control

A decline in balance control is a common problem as we age and contributes significantly to falls, particularly backward falls. Studies demonstrate that the decrease in incidental falls can be reduced by 47.5% among elderly Tai Chi Chuan practitioners. They also demonstrate better postural control than sedentary controls in simple balance tests, as well as with more sophisticated computer studies of posture. In a study of 31 subjects (mean age 68.2 ± 6.8 years), postural control was assessed by computerized posturography. The study demonstrated that there was significantly better balance performance in sway-referenced support in the Tai Chi group. Performance was significantly better for balance conditions, maximum stability, ankle strategy, and center of gravity velocity (useful in predicting falls). This investigation demonstrated that motor response and postural balance in the elderly could be improved with a committed exercise program such as Tai Chi Chuan and could help patients meet the challenge of an unforeseen fall [8].

It has been shown that Tai Chi practitioners might show better postural control, respond more quickly to an auditory command, and maintain stability better when stepping down. Thus, recovery steps are potentially more useful in this group in preventing falling when stumbling or tripping and losing balance. Those who were exercising with Tai Chi made fewer mistakes with tests that required attention resources and body control. They also had better control when standing on one leg and maintaining control when stepping down from this task [9].

Losing balance and tripping over an obstacle are frequent causes of falls. Studying and practicing Tai Chi improved the reaction to an obstacle, enabling the leg to cross the obstacle with increased leading and trailing toe clearance, and reduced variability through the crossing cycle, enabling the person to clear the obstacle safely and not fall [10].

8.3 Background on Tai Chi Chuan

Tai Chi is a martial art that originated in ancient China over 3,000 years ago during the Zhou Dynasty (1100–1221 BC). It is based on the ancient philosophy of Taoism and stresses balance. The philosophy stresses that everything is complimentary and divided into equally balanced yin and yang. Thus, the exercises are based on balance.

There are several styles, and they are each named for the persons who developed them. They include the Chen style, the Yang style (the most popular), the Wu style, and the Sun style. They each lead to health promotion, are mind-body practices, and result in efficient and functional movement patterns. Qi Tai Chi combines another ancient Chinese practice, Qigong and Tai Chi, resulting in similar health benefits.

In Tai Chi, movement is dance-like, low-impact, graceful, slow, and continuous. It is never forced, and the muscles are relaxed. The joints are not locked, and the motions are circular. The motions are named for animal actions. While participating, focus on deep breathing and on how your body is responding to the motions. Focusing without being distracted by worries and concerns is what defines meditation.

8.4 What Exactly Is Meditation?

Meditation dates to religious and philosophical practices that originated in Buddhism, Hinduism, Taoism, and Jainism. It has gained popularity worldwide as a means of self-reflection and stress reduction. While meditating, one is encouraged to find a source of focus, such as breathing. During this period, all other thoughts, worries, and distractions pass along without consternation or concern. Tai Chi involves meditation and is referred to by its Harvard Medical School proponents as meditation in motion and even medication in motion. As its popularity continues to escalate, users are encouraged to think of it as a complementary tool but never a replacement for other health practices.

8.5 Potential Benefits of Tai Chi

This holistic exercise has numerous health benefits. It increases standing balance and lower extremity strength, improves sensory awareness and execution of movements, improves the ability to coordinate muscle groups, regain muscle memory, and create neuromuscular patterns. A comprehensive analysis of 17 clinical trials in 2,365 persons with a mean age of 70.3 years has established its benefits on both cognitive function and physical performance. Its effects on cognitive function were significant, even when adjusted for physical improvement. This is important because it shows that cognitive function can improve in the aged and that Tai Chi is among the exercise activities that can accomplish this [11].

Tai chi can be adaptable and thus used with people who have disabilities, addressing the strength, endurance, flexibility, mobility, and balance impairments we commonly encounter as we age. It can follow physical therapy as a means to sustain recovery from surgery. It is a gateway to exercise and a means of boosting confidence for those who are sedentary but want to become more active and fit.

It is exercise based and nonpharmacological. It can be done as a community-based group project or alone. Tai Chi not only prevents falls but promotes social, mental, and physical health. It is already showing its value in optimizing aging and wellness. This gentle form of exercise can help maintain strength, flexibility, and balance and should be built into the routine of anyone wanting to remain fit with age.

8.6 How to Begin Tai Chi

Tai chi is relatively safe when compared with yoga, cardio-heavy programs, resistance exercises, and participatory sports like pickleball, but it requires coaching and instruction. Although it can be started at any time, those who begin early in life with Tai Chi programs gain skills, expertise, and proficiency with balance and muscle strength, two major factors the lack of which lead to falls.

As with any change in your level of exertion, it is best to clear your care with your physician. Elderly persons have different cardiovascular tolerances than those who are younger, but your endurance varies on any underlying medical condition as well as your level of training. If you have a specific fall risk that can interfere with balance, your training must be modified and coordinated with your other training programs. Your participation may be limited by joint restrictions, and adaptation by an experienced instructor may be necessary.

Finding an instructor for Tai Chi may involve some research on your part, but it will be worthwhile. There is a certification program available through the Tai Chi for Health Institute (TCHI), and you can find an instructor on their website, https://taichiforhealthinstitute.org/instructors/ . You should ask friends, your physician, or a physical therapist if they have any recommendations. Classes may be available in your community – in a community center, church, or YMCA. These will allow you to interact with others, getting both feedback and support. This is an ideal way to combat social isolation. Some patients prefer to watch YouTube videos or learn from a book.

When starting, it is important to keep your muscles loose and relaxed but be mindful of your posture. Warm up and stretch before each session. Remember to slightly bend your knees to keep your center of gravity low but do not lock your waist. Pay attention to breathing. Focusing on deep, slow, and coordinated breaths improves relaxation. Dress comfortably for maximum flexibility. Tai Chi is in fashion, and it is no surprise that Tai Chi shirts, pants, and even shoes are available for purchase, but the point is to be comfortable, wearing breathable, nonrestrictive, and loose clothing. Tai Chi shoes are also known as kung fu shoes or martial arts slippers. Your shoes should not slip, should preferably have rubber soles, and provide sufficient support to allow you to maintain your balance. The soles should be thin and minimalist. Running shoes and thick-soled walking shoes are probably unsuitable, but cross-trainer shoes may be OK.

Although the clinical evidence demonstrates that beginning Tai Chi and continuing for at least 12 weeks provides benefits, the time period should give you ample time to determine if the program is right for you. The best results are seen after a year. Like with any exercise discipline, it is a commitment, so practice regularly and be patient. Its advantage is that it is relaxing and calming and that you can progress at your own pace. The science backs it up, and while medical studies are powerful as a source of encouragement, Tai Chi will involve a serious commitment to be successful. Its focus and intervention differ from the aerobic and resistance programs that were discussed in Chap. 7, yet the results can be equally gratifying and successful in helping you maintain a good quality of life, maintain balance and strength, and prevent falls [2].

8.7 Conclusion

About 40% of older adults fall at least once yearly, greatly impacting their health, independence, and quality of life. There is evidence in the medical literature that the incidence of falls can decline with many of the interventions discussed in this book. Clinical evidence shows that Tai Chi Chuan and especially individual Tai Chi prevent falls and improve balance, muscle strength, and endurance in older adults.

Tai Chi is relatively safe, is adaptable, and can be interactive. It attracts people of all ages and levels of fitness. As it is gentle and gradual, it is very appealing to the elderly. Many senior community centers are establishing Tai Chi programs as community activities.

References

1. Liu SW, Obermeyer Z, Chang Y, Shankar KN. Frequency of ED revisits and death among older adults after a fall. Am J Emerg Med. 2015;33(8):1012–8. https://doi.org/10.1016/j.ajem.2015.04.023.
2. Li F, Harmer P, Fisher KJ, McAuley E, Chaumeton N, Eckstrom E, et al. Tai chi and fall reductions in older adults: a randomized controlled trial. J Gerontol A Biol Sci Med Sci. 2005;60(2):187–94. https://doi.org/10.1093/gerona/60.2.187.
3. Vieira ER, Palmer RC, Chaves PH. Prevention of falls in older people living in the community. BMJ. 2016;353:i1419. https://doi.org/10.1136/bmj.i1419.
4. Wayne P, Fuerst ML. The Harvard Medical School guide to tai chi. Boulder, CO: Shambhala; 2013.
5. Jones DL, Selfe TK, Wen S, Eicher JL, Wilcox S, Mancinelli C. Implementation of an evidence-based, tai Ji Quan fall prevention program in rural West Virginia churches: a RE-AIM evaluation. J Aging Phys Act. 2023;31(1):33–47. https://doi.org/10.1123/japa.2021-0274.
6. Jones DL, Acord-Vira A, Robinson MB, Talkington M, Morales AL, Pride CD, et al. Adaptation of an evidence-based, fall-prevention, tai Ji Quan exercise program for adults with traumatic brain injury: focus group results. Physiother. Theory Pract. 2022:1–9. https://doi.org/10.1080/09593985.2022.2120788.
7. Hallisy KM. Tai chi beyond balance and fall prevention: health benefits and its potential role in combatting social isolation in the aging population. Current Geriatrics Reports. 2018;7(1):37–48. https://doi.org/10.1007/s13670-018-0233-5.
8. Wong AMK, Pei Y-C, Lan C, Huang S-C, Lin Y-C, Chou S-W. Is Tai Chi Chuan effective in improving lower limb response time to prevent backward falls in the elderly? Age. 2009;31(2):163–70. https://doi.org/10.1007/s11357-009-9094-3.
9. Lu X, Siu KC, Fu SN, Hui-Chan CW, Tsang WW. Tai chi practitioners have better postural control and selective attention in stepping down with and without a concurrent auditory response task. Eur J Appl Physiol. 2013;113(8):1939–45. https://doi.org/10.1007/s00421-013-2624-9.
10. Kuo CC, Chen SC, Wang JY, Ho TJ, Lin JG, Lu TW. Effects of tai-chi Chuan practice on patterns and stability of lower limb inter-joint coordination during obstructed gait in the elderly. Front Bioeng Biotechnol. 2021;9:739722. https://doi.org/10.3389/fbioe.2021.739722.
11. Park M, Song R, Ju K, Shin JC, Seo J, Fan X, et al. Effects of tai chi and Qigong on cognitive and physical functions in older adults: systematic review, meta-analysis, and meta-regression of randomized clinical trials. BMC Geriatr. 2023;23(1):352. https://doi.org/10.1186/s12877-023-04070-2.

Appendix

Abstract The final section of this book is the appendix, because like our own, it is not essential. Here, the focus is on how muscles contract, how muscle protein synthesis is stimulated, and how muscles are degraded. It also discusses the dual role of the mammalian target of rapamycin (MTOR), both a promoter of cell growth and a destroyer of cell fragments that no longer function. This chapter will show you how caloric restriction can be associated with longevity. Since aging is the major reason for falls, this chapter will review the established hallmarks of aging with some insights into ways that the aging process might be delayed.

Keywords DNA; Cell; Muscle; Mitochondria; Autophagy; Ubiquitin; MTOR

Introduction

Falls are serious accidents that occur in association with age or debilitation. Their many causes and prevention strategies have been the focus of this book. Now, we will take a deeper dive under the hood, so to speak and will try to understand the mechanisms that are responsible for major factors in falls, the loss of muscle strength, and aging. Like an automobile, one does not have to understand all of the mechanics to drive it. Reading this chapter is not necessary to help prevent falls.

The Cell (See Fig. A.1)

The cell is the building block of an organism. Each cell is surrounded by a membrane, a layered wall that has receptors, pores, transporters, and channels that function as gates, letting in and out substances as required for cell maintenance. The

A TYPICAL CELL

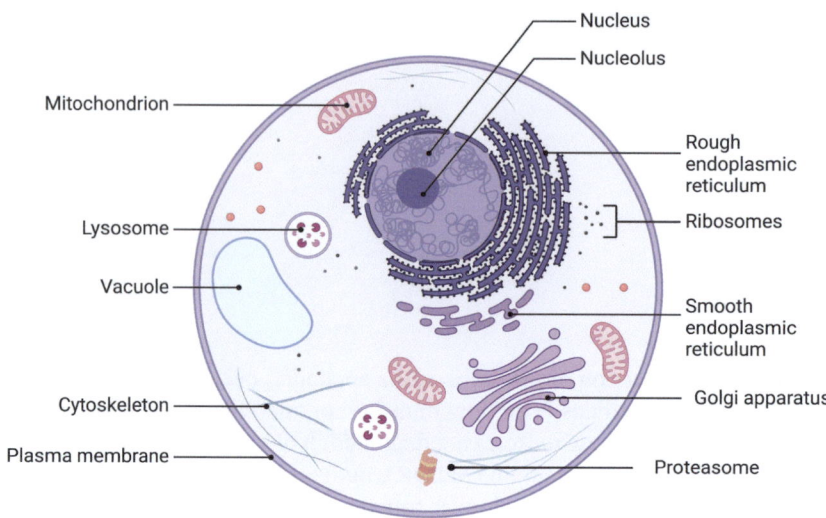

Fig. A.1 Inside the cell. Made with biorender.com

substance of the cell is called the cytoplasm, but cells are quite variable in their structure. You have already seen a very large cell – the chicken egg. Another cell, the muscle cell is loaded with bundles that contract. The cells in the body that we will be concerned with are microscopic.

Mitochondrion: This self-contained energy plant produces adenosine triphosphate (ATP), tiny molecules that pack energy in phosphate bonds. Breaking these bonds releases the energy that can drive chemical reactions. The process of making ATP requires electrons; these come from the sugars and fats that are fed into the mitochondrion, organelles (little cellular organs) that use oxygen to accept the leftover electrons that drive phosphorus coupling to ADP. Mitochondria were once bacteria. Around a billion years ago, they combined with multicellular organisms – a perfect fit. They are our house guests!!

Lysosome: This organelle can break down and reuse cellular components. During caloric restriction, signals are sent to turn on a "self-eating" system called *autophagy*. Dysfunctional organelles and other cell parts termed "cargo" are lined with a membrane called the autophagosome – the cell's equivalent of a garbage bag. This bag connects with the lysosome, literally a bag of enzymes that breaks down the cargo and recycles it.

Nucleus: The nucleus is the center of the cell and contains the genetic code – deoxyribonucleic acid or DNA. Transcription factors can select certain areas of the DNA code as they are needed. When DNA is turned on by these transcription factors, it produces messenger RNA (mRNA) that leaves the nucleus and moves the code to a ribosome.

Appendix

Endoplasmic reticulum (ER): The rough ER holds the ribosomes in place, while the smooth ER aids in housekeeping functions.

Ribosome: The ribosome is where proteins are assembled. The ribosome holds the mRNA that sends smaller transfer RNAs (tRNA) out to fetch amino acids. They will be assembled in the order specified by mRNA. The proteins will have modifications made at the ribosome level and then move to the ER lumen, where they will be folded.

Proteasome: The proteasome breaks down dysfunctional proteins. *Ubiquitins* are tiny proteins that tag the broken molecules in a three-part process that involves enzymatic activation of ubiquitin (E1) and then conjugation (E2), where the ubiquitin is conjugated to an enzyme. The third part (E3 ligase) is where the protein to be targeted is recognized, captured, and brought to the enzyme complex. The protein destined for destruction and recycling is brought to the proteasome, where it meets its fate. There are several E3 ligases in the body, each targeting different proteins.

Vacuoles: These are sacs that can store and digest toxins.

Golgi apparatus: These organelles help package lipids and proteins.

Cytoskeleton: This is a structural component of the cell that helps support it.

What Is the Day in the Life of a Cell Like? (Fig. A.2)

Glucose is fuel to the body and enters cells because of *insulin-like growth factors (IGF)* or *insulin*. When we eat sugar, the body releases insulin to help transport it into the cell. The IGF activates a receptor to receive an enzyme (tyrosine kinase)

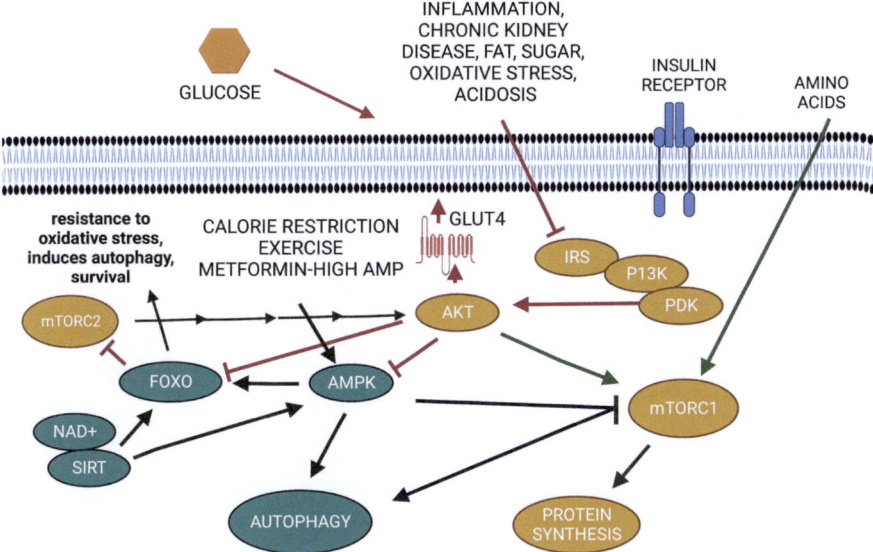

Fig. A.2 Multiple biochemical pathways control daily activity. Made with biorender.com

that works by moving the energetic phosphorus to an *insulin receptor substrate* (IRS). Many factors, including inflammation, kidney disease, high blood sugar, a diet high in saturated fats, oxidative stress, and metabolic acidosis, can weaken the IRS. When it is weakened, it causes insulin resistance. Insulin resistance plays a major role in type 2 diabetes. The factors that cause insulin resistance, and the resistance itself, lead to diabetic complications and aging.

When IRS is energized by phosphate, it serves as the docking station for another molecule, P13K (phosphoinositide-3-kinase). When PI3K is active, it turns on the PI-dependent kinase-1 (PKD), which cascades to activate ATK (named from the AKR mouse strain for thymoma), also called protein kinase B. Once activated, AKT facilitates the glucose transporter GLUT 4 to embed in the cell membrane and allow the entry of glucose.

Glucose Enters the Cell (Fig. A.3)

When glucose enters the cell, it is broken down by the process of glycolysis to pyruvate. When this glucose is broken down, it releases electrons. Hence, some ATP is produced along the sugar route to the mitochondria. This process does not require oxygen.

The pyruvates enter the mitochondria. These little organelles are specifically designed to break down fuel molecules like pyruvate through a complex chain of

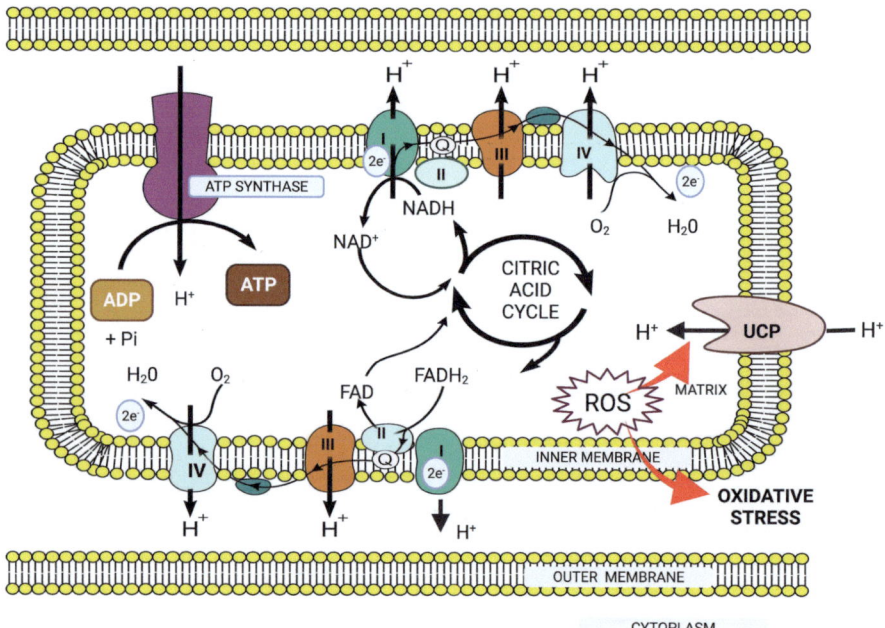

Fig. A.3 Reactions that occur inside the mitochondria

chemical reactions, known as the citric acid cycle, and use the liberated electrons to drive phosphate coupling to adenosine diphosphate (ADP), thus forming ATP. Some of the products of this chain are well-known as food supplements and multivitamins. At the end of a chain of electron-handling steps, and deep inside the mitochondria, sits oxygen. This is called respiration. Oxygen is always hungry for electrons, and it is thus necessary for the energy reactions that enable muscle contraction to occur. The by-products of respiration are water and carbon dioxide, and they allow the safe passage of electrons to the atmosphere as we exhale the carbon dioxide. The ADP, meanwhile, is released to pick up another phosphorus, and the cycle begins anew.

Oxidative Stress

Electron transfer is the key process that guides the formation of energy in the body. When a molecule has unpaired electrons, it is highly unstable and can react with and destroy adjacent tissues. This is oxidative stress. The process of antioxidation occurs when another molecule donates an electron to the unstable one without becoming unstable itself. During normal mitochondrial action, free radicals can form and can often be quickly neutralized. The environment, diet, and underlying medical conditions can also contribute to oxidative stress.

During inflammatory states, tissues may create oxidative stress purposefully to kill an invading microorganism. Although a protective mechanism, inflammation is often a consequence of a chronic disease process, and the inflammatory response is then misdirected toward the body's tissues.

AKT and mTORC

When the IGF cascade turns on AKT, it signals that the insulin fuel supply will enter the cell. This signaling shuts off the rescue protein, adenosine monophosphate kinase (AMPK), which then inhibits mTORC1. When mTORC1 is inhibited, it turns on autophagy. AMPK is a kinase (a type of enzyme) that is designed to help conserve and rescue the cell when fuel sources are low. It is activated by caloric restriction and exercise. The diabetic medication metformin and the herbal chemical berberine can also activate it. AMPK starts a housekeeping project that removes cell clutter, including dangerous fragments that can incite inflammation.

When one goes into caloric restriction, AMPK is turned on. It requires a special chemical to help handle electrons, nicotinamide riboside (NAD+), which combines with the regulator, sirtuin (SIRT), to also assist with the enzymatic process. These proteins are all associated with slowing aging. They release the forkhead transcription factor (FOXO). FOXO regulates many cellular processes, and is concerned with survival and rescue. One of its jobs is to promote the production of glucose. It is also a tumor suppressor. AMPK inhibits mTORC1 and stimulates autophagy, a process of self-digestion that essentially cleans up the cell, recycling products through the lysosome (see Fig. A.2). These survival enzymes have come to popular attention because of their potential benefits in prolonging cell survival. Much of the research that is currently being done to try to identify how aging can be slowed is centered on the benefits of SIRT, AMPK stimulation, and MTOR.

The MTOR Story (See Figs. A.4, A.5, A.6, A.7, A.8, and A.9)
In 1964, an expedition from Canada traveled to Easter Island to collect soil samples. Easter Island had been an isolated, remote volcanic island that for centuries had been home to a group of inhabitants who carved strange statues called moai from the volcanic rock. Their island was now part of Chile and plans to create a giant airstrip and increase travel threatened to change the ecology of this unique place. What was also fascinating was that inhabitants of Rapa Nui, or Easter Island, seemed to be immune from tetanus, a disease associated with horses. Rapa Nui had a large horse population, and the natives often walked barefoot. Was it possible that an antibiotic in the soil was protecting them? After analysis, tetanus was hardly even isolated in their soil, and the dirt samples were almost discarded. In 1969, the preserved soil samples were sent to Ayerst Pharmaceuticals. Ayerst worked on the project for 2 years, isolating a molecule capable of killing fungi. They named it rapamycin after the island and its people. This remarkable compound was also capable of suppressing cancer, but it appeared difficult to turn rapamycin into a commercial success, and in 1982, the project was abandoned. Ayerst moved from Montreal to Princeton, NJ. Suren Sehgal the lead scientist on the Ayerst project had confidence in this forgotten soil remnant, storing it in the family freezer next to ice cream with the label "DON'T EAT." During the move, he and his family sealed the packages with duct tape so movers would not open them. The soil remnant stayed in their freezer for the next 5 years. In 1987, when Ayerst and Wyeth merged, the new company renewed interest in rapamycin. They desired to discover a new drug that would help kidney transplant patients. Cyclosporine was the current standard of care for transplant patients, and FK506 or tacrolimus, which had a partially identical structure to rapamycin, was emerging. Rapamycin became a popular antirejection drug in 1999. Pfizer purchased Wyeth in 2009 and marketed rapamycin as Rapamune. As the pharmaceutical industry feverishly worked to identify new potential uses for rapamycin, its target emerged as central to controlling aging, autophagy, and muscle synthesis. Research on the mechanisms of how rapamycin worked revealed the discovery that the mammalian or mechanistic target of rapamycin (MTOR) has a dual function. It can promote the synthesis of proteins or it can orchestrate autophagy and move the cell into survival mode [1].

Appendix 147

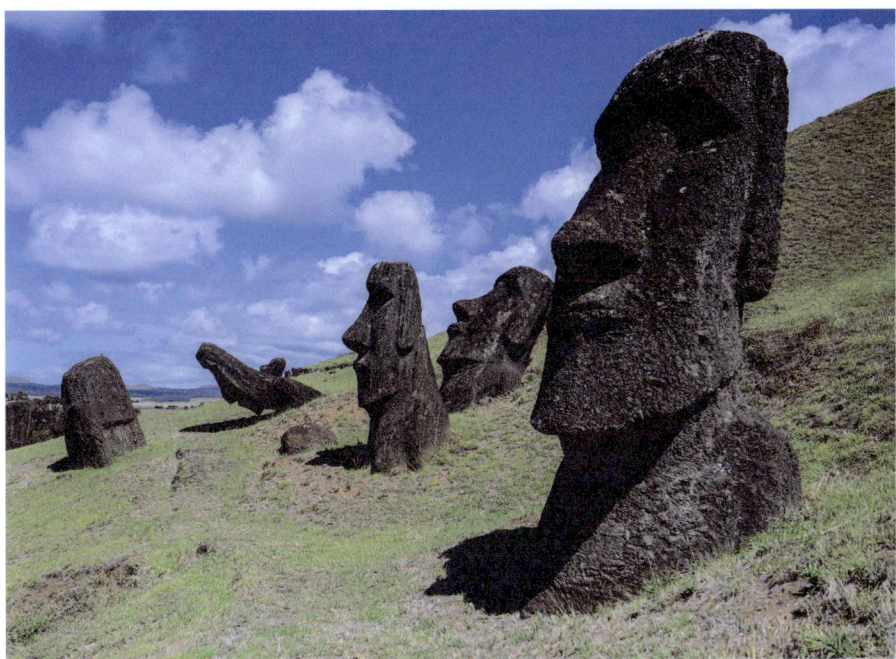

Fig. A.4 Rano Raraku on Easter Island—photograph by Stephen Fadem

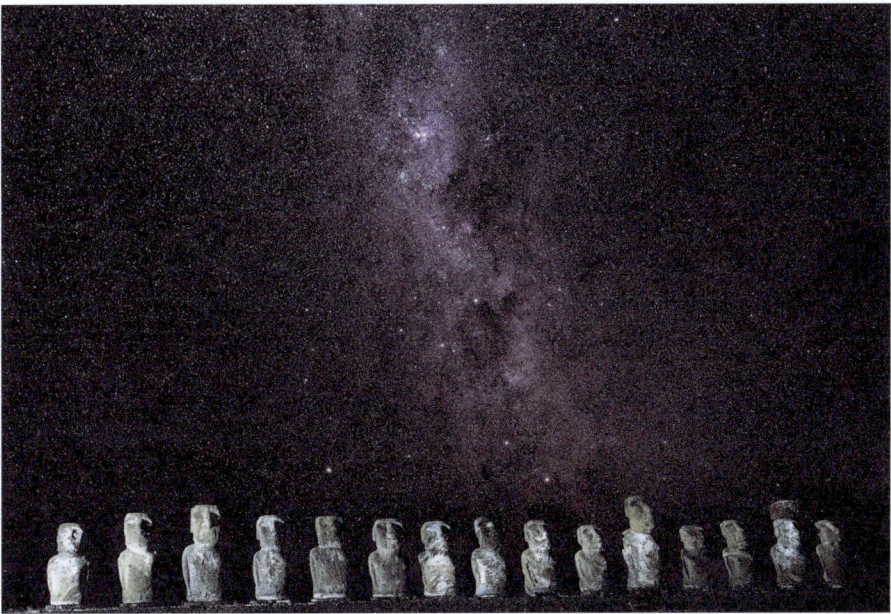

Fig. A.5 This photograph was taken at Ahu Tongariki at 1 AM on a moonless night. Easter Island is 2200 kilometers from its nearest neighbor, and the sky is so dark that the only light was the Milky Way. The 15 moai statues were illuminated with a flashlight borrowed from the hotel. Photograph by Stephen Fadem

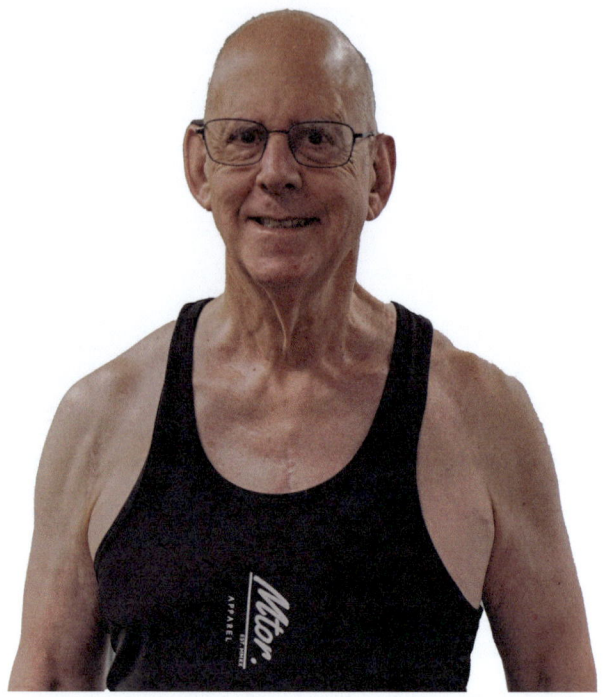

Fig. A.6 MTOR has moved to rock star status among fitness enthusiasts. It has been described as a tonic for a longer life. Photograph by Michelle (Misha) L Nguyen

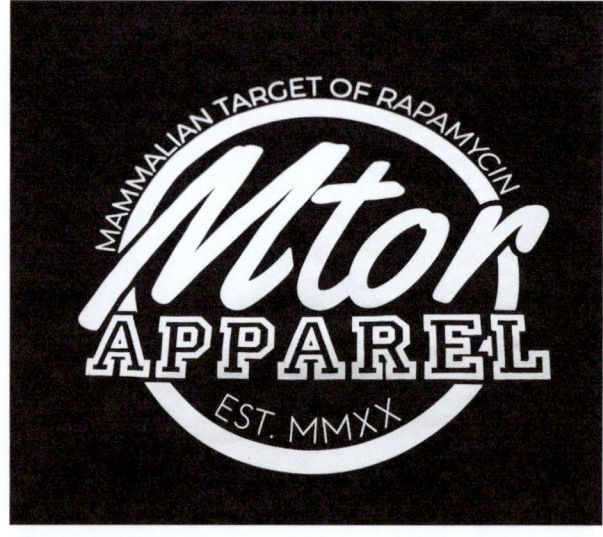

Fig. A.7 The logo of the fitness-clothing company MTOR Apparel has been inspired by the complex biochemical pathway associated with stimulating muscle growth and prolonging life. Photo by Stephen Fadem

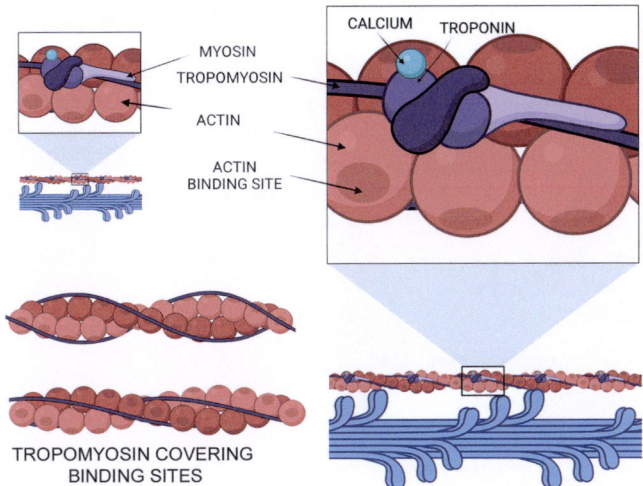

MUSCLE CONTRACTION

- You want to flex your arm
- Your brain sends a signal through the nerves to the muscle fiber.
- A chemical reaction opens channels allowing sodium to enter the muscle. This triggers the release of calcium.
- The calcium binds to a site on troponin.
- Troponin shifts tropomyosin away from the site where actin and myosin will bind.
- ATP releases energy that changes the conformation of myosin so it can bind and pull on the actin. This causes contraction.

Fig. A.8 What happens when you contract your arm. Created with biorender.com

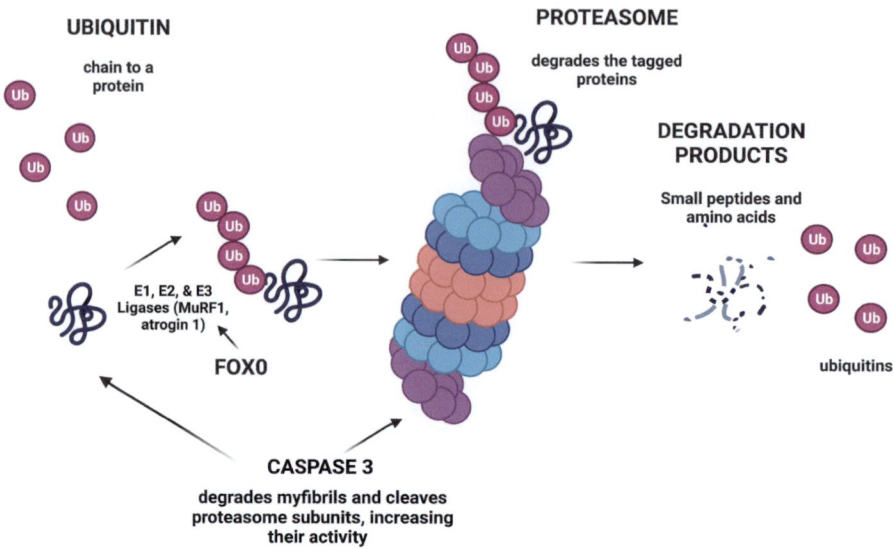

Fig. A.9 Ubiquitin tagging and proteasomal breakdown of muscle fibers

The Story of Muscles

The body contains three types of muscles: smooth muscles line blood vessels and the walls of organs like the stomach, cardiac muscle is responsible for our heart contracting, and skeletal muscle makes us mobile. Skeletal muscle contractions allow us to run, bend, flex, do gymnastics, lift weights, and keep our balance. They respond to the signals we send them. All muscles require glucose and oxygen to create energy and building blocks made up of amino acids. They also require fats and an assortment of minerals. Together, muscles are involved in chemical interactions that allow two distinct filaments, actin and myosin, to slide across each other [2, 3].

Muscles are part of an efficient system. If they feel needed (are fed properly and exercised), they grow and enlarge, but if they feel neglected, they wither. In medicine, we call this withering atrophy, which is known as sarcopenia when it concerns skeletal muscle. As we age, the signals that cause muscles to continue to grow start to drop off, but the good news is that exercise can preserve muscle function. The growth and breakdown of muscle must be in balance. When muscles grow, it is known as anabolism, but it is called catabolism when they are breaking down.

Inside of muscle cells, there are tiny organs – organelles. The nucleus of the cell sends signals known as messenger RNA (mRNA) to ribosomes. The ribosome decodes this RNA and sends transfer RNA out to find the building blocks called amino acids and neatly assemble them in a line on the ribosome to form proteins – the proteins that will make actin and myosin. Actin is a globular or spherical protein that forms a long polymer and then forms bundles. It can polymerize or depolymerize depending on the number of filaments. Thus, muscle protein synthesis plays a major role in its polymerization. Actin is also a versatile protein that is involved in many other cellular processes, i.e., mitosis. Actin is present in other cells besides human cells, even yeast. The actin has binding sites where the second protein filament – myosin – the motor protein can latch to it. It is this grabbing process that pulls the two filaments and causes contraction. The actin is sheathed by the protein, tropomyosin, that covers these grabbing sites. When calcium binds an adjacent protein, troponin, it signals the tropomyosin to rotate away and expose the grabbing or binding sites. The reaction that myosin requires to tug and pull on the actin requires energy. This energy is supplied by adenosine triphosphate (ATP) a complex that is tightly bound to phosphorus. Breaking this bond releases enough energy to force the myosin to change shape and, in the process, tug and pull against actin, shortening the muscle fiber. This is contraction [4].

We know that exercise helps preserve functional capacity in older people. So, how does bodybuilding – lifting weights against gravity – build more muscle and prevent its breakdown [5, 6]? The answer is that exercising sensitizes the body to utilize proteins to make muscles, even more so than feeding alone [7]. Resistance exercise can be done by increasing the load or by more repetitions. It does not actually matter whether one reaches the point of exhaustion to benefit, but the exercise should be intense [8].

What does amino acid intake do? Resistance exercise upregulates amino acid transcription factors along with eating and increases MTOR sensitivity to the amino acid leucine [9]. Although muscle loss accompanying starvation is protected during fasting when the ketoanalog of leucine (leucine stripped of its nitrogen) is infused into nonexercising obese subjects, it does not seem that muscle is being built but that it is not being degraded [10]. Leucine will only enhance MTOR sensitivity in the muscles that are being exercised. HMB (beta-hydroxyl beta-methyl-butyrate) is a metabolite of leucine that is used by bodybuilders. A small study in elderly men demonstrated that HMB only reduced abdominal fat mass in groups that were exercising compared to groups that were not exercising and groups not taking HMB. The authors concluded that further studies were needed to investigate this relationship [11].

High-intensity and endurance exercise improves cardiac function and blood vessels. It also increases endurance performance. Exercise in the elderly will improve insulin sensitivity and increase muscle mitochondria density. It can preserve the mitochondrial genome and in muscle. It also helps protect genes related to glucose metabolism.

Both sprinting and resistance exercises result in a strong stress response during the 3-h recovery period that follows. The central regulator of muscle protein synthesis is MTOR. It continues to combine with other factors in turning on the ribosome to make more protein. This activity is greatest when a carbohydrate beverage and post-exercise dietary protein are consumed, resulting in more muscle mass. The reactions that take place with exercise impair SMAD complexes from reaching the nucleus and stimulating myostatin, a product that breaks down muscle.

AMPK is enhanced during heavy endurance exercise, and although it blunts MTOR, its results are synergistic. Inhibiting MTOR initiates autophagy which recycles damaged proteins. MTOR blunting also allows the breakdown of damaged proteins by the ubiquitin proteasome. This is actually a quality control step. When the proteasome breaks apart damaged proteins, it degrades them to fresh amino acids that can also potentiate MTOR muscle synthesis.

When supplied with essential amino acids like leucine, found in many foods, navy beans, eggs, lentils, and oats, MTOR is turned on and promotes the proteins that make actin and myosin especially during exercise. When undergoing caloric restriction, MTOR is turned off, and a recycling housekeeping process occurs in the cell. This eliminates many potentially dangerous by-products in the cell by moving them into a giant cell waste disposal called the lysosome. Across the entire spectrum of the animal kingdom, MTOR has been central to mechanisms that prolong survival and is intensely being studied for its role in aging. Furthermore, caloric restriction potentiates AMPK, and in shutting down MTOR increases autophagy and induces FOXO. FOXO is similar to products in other eukaryotes that are associated with survival [12].

Why Does Aging Cause Muscle Breakdown?

All broken-down cellular fragments and dysfunctional proteins undergo autophagy. Even DNA that undergoes wear and tear beyond repair is removed, compromising the necessary components needed for cell maintenance. Cell function becomes maladaptive when cells can no longer process nutrients and convert them to needed biochemicals.

Concerning muscle breakdown, proteasomes contain proteases, enzymes that break down various proteins that have been tagged for destruction. The balance between protein synthesis and protein loss will determine if there are sufficient proteins to make the actin and myosin fibers that are necessary for muscles to function. Several factors upset this balance, causing profound muscle loss or sarcopenia. They include space travel, inactivity or lack of muscle use, viruses like HIV, inflammation, severe infections, starvation, cancer, metabolic acidosis, and CKD. When any of these factors are present, signals are sent to activate ubiquitin and then identify and attach activated ubiquitin to the muscle protein destined for destruction. Ubiquitins combine to build a chain carrying their prey to the proteasome. There, proteins are broken into either smaller peptides or amino acids where they can be reused.

Aging

Since a major cause of falls is old age, we should try to understand what happens when we age and identify ways to slow the aging process. No single mechanism explains aging, but there are many observations that inflammation, oxidative stress, and many chronic diseases accelerate it. These processes damage body molecules, requiring either their destruction or repair. DNA is one of the tissues that can be damaged and must be repaired.

A dominant theory is that DNA developed a survival mechanism early in evolution. A second gene would be silent when times were good so that the DNA could copy itself at will. However, when times were bad or when repair was needed, the second gene would become active, stopping reproduction and repairing the gene. This survival mechanism has existed for 4 billion years [13].

In conditions with intense exposure to oxidative stress, the mitochondria become overwhelmed and cannot effectively create ATP. Autophagy is incapable of handling the burden of damaged organelles and dysfunctional molecules. Epigenetic changes are those that occur independently of DNA. They are not inherited but strongly influence many biological processes. For instance, epigenetic mechanisms regulate the transcription mechanisms that tell DNA what to do. Several epigenetic enzymes are involved in DNA repair, but these epigenetic repair processes are insufficient when DNA damage is too extensive.

Current thinking centers around nine hallmarks of aging: (1) genomic instability leading to DNA damage, (2) shortening of the DNA endcaps or telomeres, (3) epigenetic change in the ability to repair DNA, (4) loss of autophagy and proteasome ability, (5) altered nutrient sensing – insulin resistance, (6) cell senescence, (7) stem cell exhaustion, (8) mitochondrial dysfunction, (9) altered cell signaling [14].

1. *Genomic instability:* Oxidative stress increases with aging. It is highly reactive with any cellular component and in particular destructive to mitochondria and DNA.
2. *Telomeres:* Each DNA strand has a cap or telomere that protects it from damage. Long telomeres are associated with improved longevity, but shortening is an inexorable cause of senescence. Without the protective telomere, the DNA becomes damaged and cannot function.
3. *Epigenetic modification*: The repair of DNA occurs because of epigenetic enzymes that can add two carbon vinegar-like groups (acetylation) to the support structure of the DNA called histone, stopping its action. Histone is integral for DNA wrapping and coiling. Chromatin is the combination of DNA and histone. Changes that can add simple carbon and hydrogen groups (methylation) to one of the DNA rings are also epigenetic. The addition of this carbon to the ring stops DNA. This result allows damaged DNA to be repaired. When the enzymes involved in this process are modified or overwhelmed, DNA strands go unrepaired.
4. *Proteostasis:* This refers to the impairment of the recycling mechanisms, the autophagy/lysosome path, and the ubiquitin/proteasome path. With reduced effectiveness, misfolded and dysfunctional proteins and damaged organelles do not get targeted for destruction.
5. *Altered nutrient sensing:* Sirtuins play a key role, along with NAD+ and caloric restriction, in inhibiting mTOR and enabling autophagy. IGF-1 signaling blocks AMPK. This mechanism is preserved across evolution; altered gene homologs

of the IGF-1 receptor, *daf*-2, and PI3K, *age*-1, are associated with a longer life span in *C. elegans*. Activating the homolog of FOXO, DAF-16, also increases longevity.
6. *Cellular senescence:* This occurs when cellular functions are disrupted. As the cell becomes worn, it cannot repair itself. Altered telomeres lead to dysfunctional DNA that cannot send RNA codes to ribosomes. This leads to the eventual breakdown of the biological processes the cell must rely on – mitochondria cannot create energy, and the cell's ability to fend off stress is diminished. Without these protections, the cell becomes senescent and dies.
7. *Stem cell exhaustion:* Muscles, blood vessels, and the immune system are among the body tissues that rely on stem cells throughout our life. As aging occurs, the stem cell numbers decrease and the tissues that rely on them cannot be restored.
8. *Mitochrondrial dysfunction*: As the cell ages, the mitochondria cannot generate energy, compromising all biochemical reactions that depend upon ATP.
9. *Altered cellular communication*: As cells age, the immune system starts to fail. Neurons also start to fail.

Fortunately, several steps can be taken that show promise in slowing the aging process:

- Eat healthy but not too much – Sirtuins play a vital role in epigenetic repair, but the production of these enzymes declines with age, as does the NAD+ that works alongside the sirtuins to activate AMPK. Many of the cofactors that mitochondria rely on are well-known vitamins. Foods high in flavonoids, like fruits and vegetables, may help replenish some of the nutrients vital for cellular function. Other foods that have a high oxidation potential place an extra burden on the epigenetic mechanisms that repair DNA. Restricting calories turns on ancient mechanisms like AMPK, vital in blocking MTOR and stimulating autophagy, the housekeeping service of the cell. Meanwhile, eating foods rich in amino acids like leucine – eggs, navy beans, and lentils for example – can turn on MTOR when accompanied by resistance exercise, helping to restore skeletal muscle.
- Do not smoke. While popular in the early part of the past century, countless studies have demonstrated the dangers of smoking at a cellular level.
- Exercise – Each step to help reduce the fall risk can also help stall aging. Mental and cardiovascular function improves with exercise. Exercise helps rebuild the muscle lost with the aging process.
- Drug therapy to prevent aging, maintain stem cells, and stop the clock are unfortunately in the future and perhaps our current reach. Clinical trials must demonstrate that they are both safe and effective before they can be recommended. The pipeline for drug therapy is promising. For instance, age-related macular degeneration (AMD) is apparently related to mitochondrial damage and oxidative stress. The AREDS2 trial has demonstrated that AMD can be delayed using well-known and established vitamins that one can purchase over the counter. Several clinical trials are in progress that show promise [15]. AMD is a window into the aging process itself, and it makes sense that several of the maneuvers taken to prevent its worsening will also impact other side effects of aging [16].

- NAD+ precursors, mitochondrial support supplements, sirtuin-containing foods, AMPK activators like metformin and berberine, antioxidants like N-acetyl-cysteine, flavonoids, and sirtfoods like dark chocolate are readily available. However, it is always best to rely on clinical trial-based evidence and beware of bold statements made without factual backup [17–19].

Conclusion

This chapter discusses how muscles contract, how cells age, and how caloric restriction can block an almost forgotten chemical found on Easter Island and unlock the secrets to longevity. While still far from the Fountain of Youth, research into aging shows much promise. We must build muscle strength to avoid falls, particularly in our lower bodies and core. This chapter helps explain how exercise stimulates muscle growth and how muscles are degraded. It ends with a discussion on the hallmarks of aging, the major factor in falls.

References

Halford B. Rapamycin's secrets unearthed. Chem Eng News. 2016;94:29.

Schiaffino S, Dyar KA, Ciciliot S, Blaauw B, Sandri M. Mechanisms regulating skeletal muscle growth and atrophy. FEBS J. 2013;280(17):4294–314. https://doi.org/10.1111/febs.12253.

Bodine SC, Stitt TN, Gonzalez M, Kline WO, Stover GL, Bauerlein R, et al. Akt/mTOR pathway is a crucial regulator of skeletal muscle hypertrophy and can prevent muscle atrophy in vivo. Nat Cell Biol. 2001;3(11):1014–9. https://doi.org/10.1038/ncb1101-1014.

Lehman W, Craig R, Vibert P. Ca(2+)-induced tropomyosin movement in limulus thin filaments revealed by three-dimensional reconstruction. Nature. 1994;368(6466):65–7. https://doi.org/10.1038/368065a0.

Van Roie E, Walker S, Van Driessche S, Delabastita T, Vanwanseele B, Delecluse C. An age-adapted plyometric exercise program improves dynamic strength, jump performance and functional capacity in older men either similarly or more than traditional resistance training. PLoS One. 2020;15(8):e0237921. https://doi.org/10.1371/journal.pone.0237921.

Smith JAB, Murach KA, Dyar KA, Zierath JR. Exercise metabolism and adaptation in skeletal muscle. Nat Rev Mol Cell Biol. 2023; https://doi.org/10.1038/s41580-023-00606-x.

Phillips SM. The impact of protein quality on the promotion of resistance exercise-induced changes in muscle mass. Nutr Metab (Lond). 2016;13(1):64. https://doi.org/10.1186/s12986-016-0124-8.

Refalo MC, Helms ER, Trexler ET, Hamilton DL, Fyfe JJ. Influence of resistance training proximity-to-failure on skeletal muscle hypertrophy: a systematic review with meta-analysis. Sports Med. 2023;53(3):649–65. https://doi.org/10.1007/s40279-022-01784-y.

D'Hulst G, Masschelein E, De Bock K. Resistance exercise enhances long-term mTORC1 sensitivity to leucine. Mol Metab. 2022;66:101615. https://doi.org/10.1016/j.molmet.2022.101615.

Mitch WE, Walser M, Sapir DG. Nitrogen sparing induced by leucine compared with that induced by its keto analogue, alpha-ketoisocaproate, in fasting obese man. J Clin Invest. 1981;67(2):553–62. https://doi.org/10.1172/jci110066.

Stout JR, Fukuda DH, Kendall KL, Smith-Ryan AE, Moon JR, Hoffman JR. β-Hydroxy-β-methylbutyrate (HMB) supplementation and resistance exercise significantly reduce abdominal adiposity in healthy elderly men. Exp Gerontol. 2015;64:33–4. https://doi.org/10.1016/j.exger.2015.02.012.

Masters TA, Kendrick-Jones J, Buss F. Myosins: domain organisation, motor properties, physiological roles and cellular functions. Handb Exp Pharmacol. 2017;235:77–122. https://doi.org/10.1007/164_2016_29.

Mishra S, Raval M, Kachhawaha AS, Tiwari BS, Tiwari AK. Aging: epigenetic modifications. Prog Mol Biol Transl Sci. 2023;197:171–209. https://doi.org/10.1016/bs.pmbts.2023.02.002.

López-Otín C, Blasco MA, Partridge L, Serrano M, Kroemer G. The hallmarks of aging. Cell. 2013;153(6):1194–217. https://doi.org/10.1016/j.cell.2013.05.039.

Chew EY, Clemons TE, Agrón E, Domalpally A, Keenan TDL, Vitale S, et al. Long-term outcomes of adding lutein/zeaxanthin and ω-3 fatty acids to the AREDS supplements on age-related macular degeneration progression: AREDS2 report 28. JAMA Ophthalmol. 2022;140(7):692–8. https://doi.org/10.1001/jamaophthalmol.2022.1640.

Lenin RR, Koh YH, Zhang Z, Yeo YZ, Parikh BH, Seah I, et al. Dysfunctional autophagy, Proteostasis, and mitochondria as a prelude to age-related macular degeneration. Int J Mol Sci. 2023;24(10) https://doi.org/10.3390/ijms24108763.

Chowdhury SG, Misra S, Karmakar P. Understanding the impact of obesity on ageing in the radiance of DNA metabolism. J Nutr Health Aging. 2023;27(5):314–28. https://doi.org/10.1007/s12603-023-1912-1.

Imai S, Guarente L. NAD+ and sirtuins in aging and disease. Trends Cell Biol. 2014;24(8):464–71. https://doi.org/10.1016/j.tcb.2014.04.002.

Kida Y, Goligorsky MS. Sirtuins, cell senescence, and vascular aging. Can J Cardiol. 2016;32(5):634–41. https://doi.org/10.1016/j.cjca.2015.11.022.

Index

A
Ablation therapy, 28
Acute myocardial infarction, 29
Adenosine diphosphate (ADP), 145
Adipokines, 26
Age-related falls, 82
Agility, 124
Aging, 125
Aging process, 152, 154, 155
AKT, 145
Altered cellular communication, 154
Altered nutrient sensing, 153
Alzheimer's disease, 13
AMD, 154
American College of Cardiology, 24
American Heart Association (AHA), 27
American Heart Association guidelines, 24
Americans with Disabilities Act (ADA) website, 47
Amino acid intake, 151
AMPK, 145, 152
Anticholinergics, 87
Antioxidation, 145
Arthritis, 86
Arthritis and peripheral neuropathy, 30
Assistive devices, 53, 54, 106–108, 114
ATP, 144
Atrial clot formation, 28
Atrial fibrillation, 27, 28
Autophagy, 152, 153

B
Balance, 31, 41, 129–130
Balance control, 136
Balance disorders, 42
Balance Exercises, 125
Balance losses, 49
Balance system in the brain, 42
Balanced Rock, 113
Berg Balance Scale (BBS), 136
Biochemical pathways control daily activity, 143
Biomarkers, 28
Blood distribution in the body, 55
Blunt force of a sudden impact, 63
Bone cells, 66
Bone formation, 33
Bone formation and mineralization, 33
Bone loss, 89
Bone mineral density test (BMD), 33
Bone-making proteins, 32
Brain concussion, 62
Brain contusion, 63

C
Calcified organisms, 33
Calcium, 8
Cancellous or trabecular bone, 66
Cancer and chronic conditions, 30
Cardiac biomarkers, 28–34

Carpeting, 49
CDC, 73
Cell, 141
Cell like
　life, 143–144
Cellular senescence, 154
Centers for Disease Control and Prevention
　(CDC), 72
Chronic heart disease, 27
Chronic Illnesses and Disorders, 20–21
　age, 20
　genetic composition, 21
Chronic kidney disease, 83–84
Chronic obstructive pulmonary disease
　(COPD), 29
Chronic traumatic encephalopathy
　(CTL), 15, 63
Circadian rhythm, 29
Coefficient of friction (COF) or resistance, 46
Cognitive behavioral therapy, 29
Cognitive decline, 75–81
Comorbidities, 82
Competitive sport, 2
Congestive heart failure, 27, 84–85
Continuous glucose monitoring (CGM), 25
Controlling acidosis, 22
Core, 126, 127
COVID-19 pandemic, 7, 28
Cytoskeleton, 143

D
Dementia, 13, 78–81
Demineralized bone, 65
Diabetes, 6, 8, 83, 84
Diabetes mellitus, 25
Diabetic retinopathy, 86
Diabetic therapy, 19
Dialysis, 5, 83
Dialysis procedure, 5, 34
Diuretics and blood pressure medications, 18
DNA, 9
Dominant theory, 153
Drug therapy, 154
Dynamic coefficient of friction
　(DCOF), 46, 97
Dynamic COF (DCOF), 46

E
Electron transfer, 145
Endoplasmic reticulum (ER), 143
Endurance and Fitness, 124

English Longitudinal Study of Aging, 31
Environmental fall hazards, 41, 79
Epigenetic modification, 153
Excessive daytime sleeping, 29
Exercise, 89, 90, 117, 132
Extradural (also known as epidural)
　hematoma, 64
Eye injuries, 131

F
Fall after a stroke, 12
Fall-associated fractures in the elderly, 55
Falling during daily activities, 3
Falling on the stairs, 44
Fall-risk-inducing drugs (FRIDS), 81
Falls
　mechanical, 3
　non-mechanical, 3
　precautions, 2
Falls after a stroke, 12
Falls on stairs or secondary to tripping, 67
Fatigue and exhaustion, 56, 109
Femoral shaft fractures, 68
Fitness and Mobility Exercise (FAME)
　Program, 78, 117
Fitness and Mobility Exercise (FAME)
　Program for stroke, 77, 122
Fitness snacks, 125, 130
Floor surfaces, 45
Foot disorders, 88–89
Forearm fractures, 68
Forkhead transcription factor (FOXO), 145
Forward momentum, 100
4-stage balance test, 74
FOXO, 152
Fracture risk reduction and improved skeletal
　health in diabetes, 26
Fractures, 65
Frailty, 6, 9, 10, 75
Frailty and falls, 11
FRIDS, 16
Fried's classification, 10
Frontotemporal Dementia (FTD), 14
Furosemide, 82

G
Gait disorders, 31
Gait strength and balance, 72, 73
Gait technique, 87
Genomic instability, 153
Glucagon-like peptide (GLP-1), 26

Index

Glucose, 143
Glucose management indicator (GMI) based on clinical trials, 19
Glycolysis, 144
Golgi apparatus, 143
Gravity on bone, 10
Group activities, 133
Gym activities, 2

H
Handrails, 45
Harvard Special Health Report, 135
HbA1C, 19, 20
Heart failure, 27
Heart rate reserve (HRR), 78
Hematomas, 63–65
High-intensity and endurance exercise, 151
Hiking, 56
Hip fractures, 67–68
HMB (beta-hydroxyl beta-methyl-butyrate), 151
Hypertension, 8, 24–25, 84
Hypoglycemia, 19, 26

I
Immobility, 10
Inactivity, 131
Individual *vs* Traditional Tai Chi, 135, 136
Individualized Tai Chi (iTC), 135
Inflammation, 7, 145
Insulin, 143
Insulin receptor substrate (IRS), 144
Insulin-like growth factors (IGF), 143

J
Jefferson Memorial, 98
Jutting objects, 49, 50

K
KDIGO Guidelines, 19
Kidney disease, 7, 21, 22
    weak bones
        falls and fractures, 23

L
Ladder-related accidents, 103
Lateral stability, 132
Lewy Body Dementia (LBD), 13

Lighting and depth perception, 51
Loneliness and social isolation, 136
Losing balance and tripping over an obstacle, 137
Lower body exercises, 127
Lysosome, 142

M
Maladaptive responses associated with kidney disease and hypertension, 6
Maximum target heart rate (MTHR), 78, 122
Mechanical (environmental) reasons for falls, 43, 44
Mechanical falls, 3, 5
    environmental, 41
    external factors, 41
    external floor and poor decks, 46
    eyesight, 43
    falling backward from standing position, 46
    guardrail safety, 58
    inner ear, 42
    ladder accidents, 49–51
    loss of balance, 47
    prevention of
        bath seats, 99
        blood pressure, 108
        blood pressure medications and dehydration, 108
        bump cap, 110, 111
        communication, 108
        cowboy hats, 111
        damaged ladders, 103
        falls downstairs, 96
        footwear, 109, 110
        furniture placement, 105
        grab bars, 99, 100
        grabbers, 104
        handrails, 97
        hats or helmets, 110
        headlamp, 113
        hiking outdoors, 114
        hiking sticks, 109
        jutting objects, 102
        jutting objects like cabinet doors, 102
        ladder accidents, 103
        losing balance and falling on stairs, 96
        muscle memory for recovery, 100
        nightlights, 107
        parking blocks, 100
        planning and construction, 95
        proper footwear, 114

Mechanical falls (*cont.*)
    proper planning, 95
    rugs and carpets wrinkle free, 102–103
    slippery surfaces, 97, 99
    small-area rugs, 102
    swing motion, 103
    ultraviolet light waves, 110
    uneven surfaces and small steps, 99
    up or down stairs, 96
    walking sticks, 109
    wall-to-wall carpets, 102
    washing devices for safety and convenience, 99
    wearing sun protection, 110
  Rocks and edges, 57
  rugs and carpets, 49
  specially padded exercise shorts, 80
  standing rapidly from a lying or sitting position, 55
  sudden loss of balance, 41
  swaying, 43
  uneven or jutting surfaces, 48
Medical assistance in national or state parks, 56
Medicare Claims, 25
Meditation, 137
Melatonin, 29
Minor trauma, 64
Mitochondria, 142
Mitochondrion, 142
Mitochrondrial dysfunction, 154
MTOR, 148
MTOR blunting, 152
MTOR STORY, 146
mTORC1, 145
Muscle breakdown, 152
Muscle breakdown and production, 32
Muscle weakness, 87
Muscles, types of, 150, 151

N

National Center for Injury Prevention and Control (NCIPC), 118
National Institute for Occupational Safety and Health (NIOSH), 49–51
National Safety Council, 41
Neighboring proteins, 33
Neurologic deficit, 75–81
Nicotinamide riboside (NAD+), 145
Nightlights, 51, 53, 54
NIOSH angle measuring tool, 103
Nocturia, 86
Non-mechanical falls, 3, 5, 34
Nucleic acids, 9
Nucleus, 142
Nutrition and vitamin Supplements, 80

O

Obesity, 8
Obstructive sleep apnea, 85
Opioids, 17, 18
Orthostatic hypotension, 34
Orthostatic or postural hypotension, 28, 55
Osteoclasts, 32, 65
Osteoporosis, 33, 65, 89
Osteosarcopenia, 33
Otago Balance Exercises, 120, 121
Otago Exercise Program (OEP), 76, 77, 88, 117, 122
Otago Strength exercises, 119
OTC medications, 15, 16
Oxidative stress, 7, 145, 153
Oxygen, 7

P

P13K (phosphoinositide-3-kinase), 144
Pain and muscle weakness, 86
Parkinsonian gait, 31
Participation in play, 2
Peripheral neuropathy, 30, 88–89
Phosphate coupling, 145
Phosphorus, 22
PI-dependent kinase-1 (PKD), 144
Pickleball, 131–133
Plan of care, 90
Polypharmacy, 20
Postural control, 44, 136
Postural hypotension, 28, 31, 85
Prefrail, 10
Proprioception, 41, 43, 86
Proprioception or sense of position, 43
Proteasome, 143, 152
Protein synthesis, 152
Proteostasis, 153
Pumping motion, 24

R

Randomized trials, 75
Reacher grabber, 51, 52
Recovery Step Exercises, 130

Resistance exercise, 151
Ribosome, 143
RNA, 9
Rugs, 49
Runx2, 32

S
Sarcopenia, 32, 88
Screening Tool of Older Persons; Potentially Inappropriate Prescriptions (STOPP), 82
Sedatives, 18
Sedatives and falls, 16
Selective serotonin reuptake inhibitors (SSRIs), 81
Self-directed home exercises, 122
Serum albumin, 6
Severe head injury, 63
SGLT-2 inhibitors, 26
Sirtuin (SIRT), 145, 153
Skeletal fractures, 23
Skull fractures, 63
Sleep Disorders and Falls, 29
Smartphones, 81
Soccer, 131–132
Social isolation and depression, 136
Sodium-glucose cotransporter-2 (SGLT-2) inhibitors, 26
Spinal Cord Injuries, 65
Spongy trabecular or cancellous bone, 65
SPRINT (Systolic Blood Pressure Intervention Trial), 25
Sprinting and resistance exercises, 151
STEADI, 72
Stem cell exhaustion, 154
Strength, 123
Strengthening muscles, 77
Stretching, 125, 126
Strokes, 11, 28
Structural heart disease, 27
Subarachnoid hemorrhage, 65
Subdural hematomas, 64
Sun protection, 112
Surprise question (SQ), 10
Syncope, 84

T
Tai chi, 3, 138, 139
Tai Chi Chuan (tTC), 135, 137
Tai Chi for Health Institute (TCHI), 139
Tai-chi-like movements, 78
Tai Chi practitioners, 137
Tai Chi programs, 135
Telomere shortening, 9
Telomeres, 153
Timed Up & Go, 72
Timed up-and-go (TUG) test, 136
Tissue support, Elginerpetons, 22, 23
Traditional Tai Chi programs (tTC), 135, 136
Traumatic brain injury (TBI), 62
Tripping, 51
Troponin, 28

U
Ubiquitin, 143, 150, 152

V
Vacuoles, 143
Vascular dementia, 14
Vertebral fractures, 66, 67
Vertigo, 88
Vision, 105
Visual impairment, 31
Vitamin D deficiency, 6, 32, 33
Volume control through maintaining adequate hydration, 90
Volume related disorders, 34, 89–90

W
Watchman implant, 28
Water pills, 82
Wheelchair accidents, 107
Wheelchair safety, 55
Wheelchair transfer techniques, 108

Z
Zero COF rating, 46

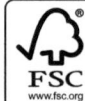

MIX
Papier aus verantwortungsvollen Quellen
Paper from responsible sources
FSC® C105338

If you have any concerns about our products,
you can contact us on
ProductSafety@springernature.com

In case Publisher is established outside the EU,
the EU authorized representative is:
**Springer Nature Customer Service Center GmbH
Europaplatz 3, 69115 Heidelberg, Germany**

Printed by Libri Plureos GmbH
in Hamburg, Germany